The Weight & Wellness Way Cookbook and Nutrition Guide.

3rd Edition. Published by: Nutritional Weight & Wellness, Inc.®
Previously published in 2014
Paintings by Cal De Reyuter

ISBN 978-0-578-86796-0

To order additional copies contact:

Nutritional Weight & Wellness, Inc.
45 Snelling Avenue North
St. Paul, MN 55104
651-699-3438 | weightandwellness.com

Table of Contents

Table of Contents

Table of Contents

Soups, Salads & Dressings

Soups

Salads

Sauces & Dressings

Table of Contents

Acknowledgements

Let me say thank you to all the nutrition educators, dietitians, nutritionists, graphic designers, writers, editors, staff, professional and home cooks, and clients who contributed their time, talents and ideas to the Weight & Wellness Way Cookbook. This would not have been possible without your help and was truly a team effort; so thank you again.

Darlene

Preface

How would you like to enjoy a better quality of life and protect your health just by making good nutrition part of your everyday routine? Years of experience have taught me that most people genuinely want to eat healthy foods, but are unsure about what is healthy. Unfortunately, the lack of accurate nutrition information and misinformation, what I call "TV nutrition" often cause people to choose processed foods over real foods.

To reverse the current health crisis, I believe that we must return to eating real food and taking the time to visit and discuss the day over a meal. Our work ethic has overshadowed the value we place on healthy food and nutrition. We skip breakfast, work through lunch, and get a "grab and go" dinner. Texting, Facebook and Instagram posts have replaced mealtime conversation. Food has become a commodity, not a way to nourish our bodies and brains. A recent survey indicated that most people want larger portions and are less concerned with taste and quality. Skipping meals and eating on the run create a feeding frenzy that can result in overeating, obesity, cholesterol problems, diabetes, low moods and aching bodies. I hope to inspire you to respect the value of good quality food. You will then become aware of the powerful, healing nature of real food.

After counseling and educating thousands of clients about nutrition for over 30 years, I have observed that most of us are not gourmet chefs; we are simply cooks who have been called upon to feed our families. We want recipes that contain relatively few ingredients and easy-to-follow directions. Most of us are willing to follow a plan that is manageable and produces the results we desire.

My goal for The Weight & Wellness Way Cookbook is to provide a balanced eating plan that is so easy to follow and so valuable to your health that it becomes your new way of life. Whether you are cooking for a large family or just for yourself, these nutritious recipes can guide you to a happier, healthier life—one you may never have thought possible.

Darlene Kvist, M.S., C.N.S., L.N.

Introduction

Nutritional Weight & Wellness created The Weight & Wellness Way with your health and well-being in mind. This simple guide for healthy eating fits most lifestyles from singles to families, and most health concerns. We know how busy you are, so we created delicious recipes that are easy to prepare with step-by-step instructions. We recognize that while some of us are creative cooks, most of us are not chefs and simply want to put healthy, tasty meals on our tables.

To eat healthy foods, you need to plan, shop and prepare good food. We designed the recipes in this book to make food and eating an enjoyable part of your day—neither an afterthought nor an obsession. Because we understand the critical role nutrition plays in health, we want to give you the tools to make healthy eating a part of your everyday routine. Once you begin to experience the benefits, such as increased energy, stable moods, fewer cravings, less pain and inflammation, and a healthy weight, we know you will find your own reasons to make healthy eating a priority.

Why was the Weight & Wellness Way created?

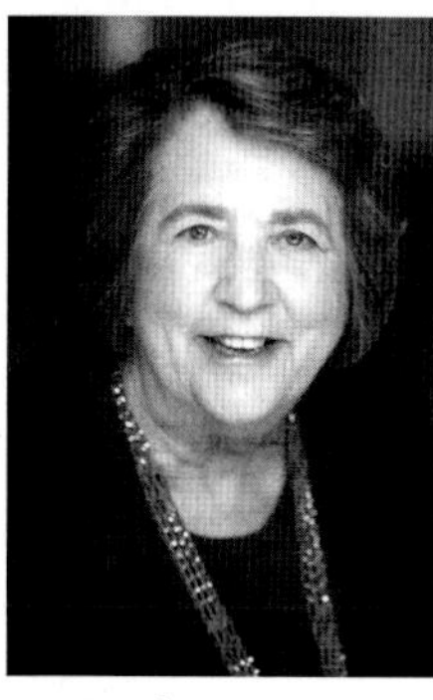

Darlene Kvist
MS, CNS, LN

Darlene Kvist, licensed nutritionist and founder of Nutritional Weight & Wellness, became alarmed by the increasing prevalence and severity of health problems in her clients. Growing up on a farm, Darlene knew how good she felt eating animal protein, lots of vegetables and real butter. She realized that most of her clients no longer ate real foods. They ate mostly processed foods that were full of additives and preservatives. Along with others in the nutrition field who expressed concern about the long-term health effects of these chemicals, Darlene made the association between the change in the American diet and the corresponding deterioration of health. She looked beyond "the party line" for better answers for creating good health. Extensive research, clinical observations, sound nutrition principles and intuition all factored into the creation of the Weight & Wellness Way.

Wanting to offer people a better option, Darlene created a simple eating plan with real food that was nutrient based, balanced blood sugar throughout the day and worked for the entire family. Using this approach, she helped clients rebuild their health and their lives with sound nutrition principles.

After counseling hundreds of people with health needs, Darlene was amazed by the lack of knowledge and understanding that many people have about how the foods they eat affect their health. People often mistake dieting for healthy eating. They have a fear of eating healthy fats, but often overeat processed junk food, fast food or fat free foods.

Many people feel their eating is out of control, and they are exhausted, irritable and have digestive problems. Often what drives people to see a nutritionist is a desire to lose weight. However, when clients change their eating and follow a healthy plan, they discover that they have more energy, less pain, and they lose weight. Weight loss alone never motivates people sufficiently to stay on a healthy eating plan. When people think of a diet, they always want to cheat. However, when people choose foods to help reduce their pain and inflammation or increase their energy, they see the benefits of good nutrition and no longer view healthy eating as a burden.

Stop thinking diet; start thinking health!

The Weight & Wellness Way protects blood vessels, supports the cartilage in joints, stabilizes blood sugar, promotes positive thoughts and balances hormones. When people eat this way, they often find that their focus, energy and thought patterns change. We have seen conditions ranging from MS, colitis and Crohn's disease go into remission for years. People experience relief from fibromyalgia, acne clears, and cancer patients live longer than predicted. These amazing health transformations occur when people stop thinking "diet" and start thinking "health".

How do these transformations come about? By eating real food: adequate animal protein, mostly vegetable carbohydrates and healthy fats in balance. Your body, perhaps for the first time, will have the right balance of nutrients to function well. You will see and feel the difference.

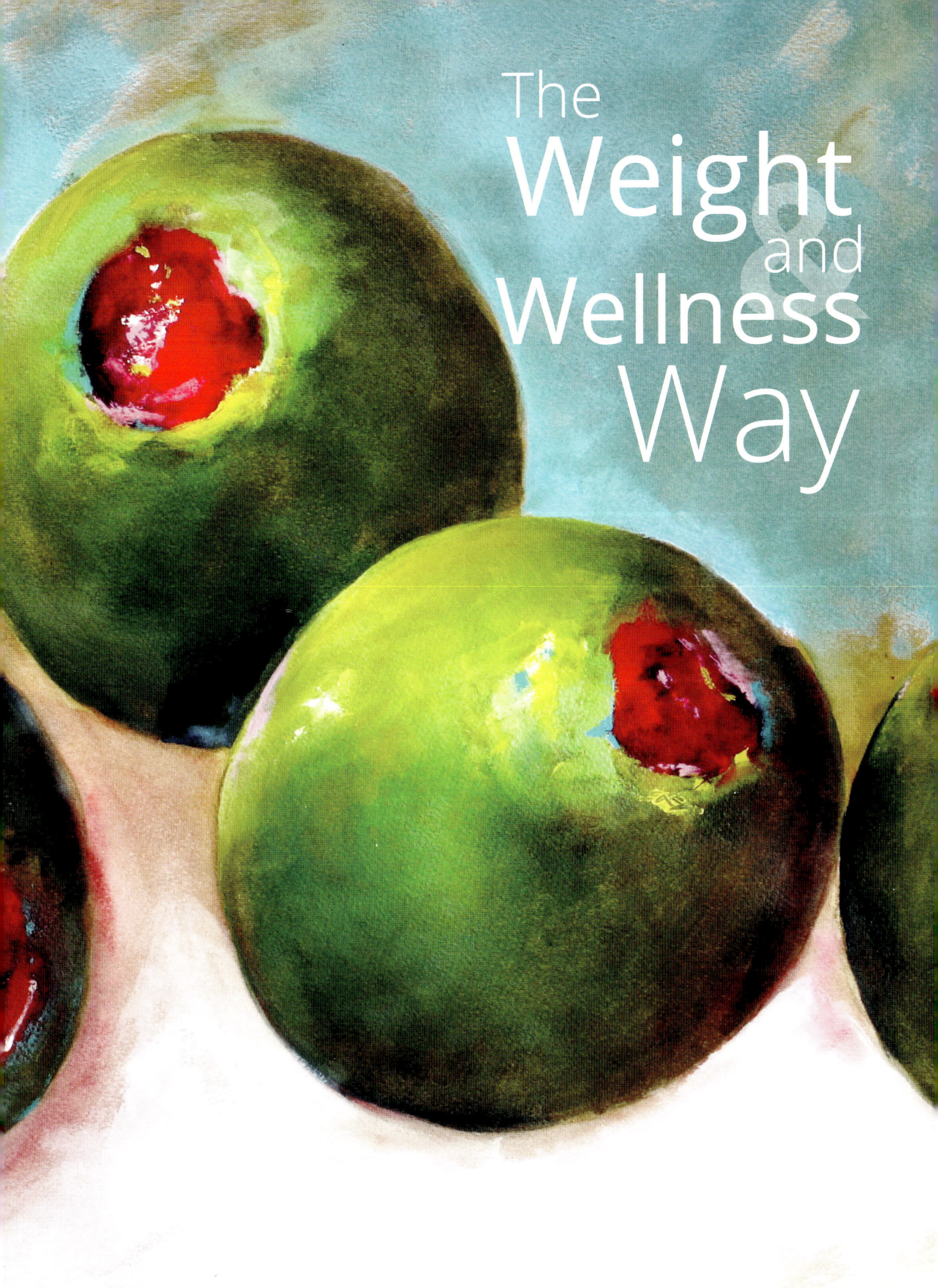
The
Weight
&
and
Wellness
Way

Start Your Day With A Wellness Check

Each day, take a few moments to check in with yourself. This is a good way to keep track of whether the changes you are making are improving your health.

Rate your energy

tired good energy feeling great

Determine your mood level

negative positive positive & productive

Evaluate how rested you are

tired restored energetic

Rate your pain level

high pain moderate pain no pain

The Weight & Wellness Way

The Weight & Wellness Way eating plan is scientifically based, clinically proven and easy to follow. This plan focuses on nutrients, not calories. You will find it simple (no counting), flexible and doable. Because you will eat plenty of food, you will not go hungry, feel deprived or have cravings! The Weight & Wellness Way balances protein, carbohydrates and fats for health and well-being.

Health benefits

- Creates energy
- Provides mental focus
- Supports well-being
- Decreases inflammation
- Helps balance blood sugar
- Assists in maintaining a healthy weight

Best of all, it works for most people!

What makes the Weight & Wellness Way different?

First and foremost, this eating plan is based on nutrients from real foods, not man-made, processed foods. The ingredients come from Mother Nature, not from a test tube or food kitchen lab. (We promise no bad fats or high fructose corn syrup in these recipes.) Another underlying principle of the Weight & Wellness Way is that balancing your blood sugar helps you experience better health, moods, energy and metabolism. This eating plan provides real foods and ample fiber with a balance of protein, carbohydrates and fat. The Weight & Wellness Way can work for everyone in your family, regardless of health conditions.

How does it work?

The Weight & Wellness Way is easy to follow whether you are eating at home, dining out, traveling, at school or at work. Singles and families find it workable as do people at all ages and stages of life.

You will learn how to balance meals and snacks throughout the day. The Weight & Wellness Way also includes behavioral and self-care strategies to help you make healthy eating part of your daily routine. By eating protein, carbohydrates and healthy fats five to six times per day, you keep your blood sugar balanced. You will find that the Weight & Wellness Way of eating leaves you energized, satisfied, alert and thinking positive thoughts. Stable blood sugar also results in less inflammation, fewer cravings and better metabolism.

The Weight & Wellness Way Eating Plan

Ready to start? It's simple. Just pick a **protein**, **carbohydrate** and **fat** from the lists that follow for every meal and snack and you will be eating the Weight & Wellness Way.

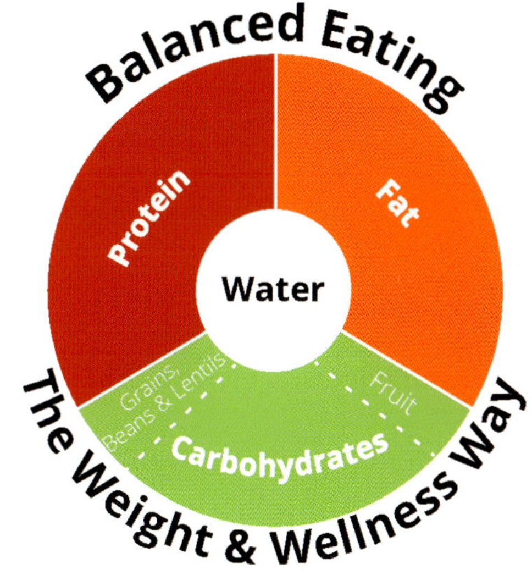

Carbohydrates

The most nutrient-dense carbohydrates are vegetables, vegetables and more vegetables. Consider vegetables as your main carbohydrate selection, whole grains as a side dish and fruit as your dessert. Include a wide selection of colors, tastes and textures, both raw and cooked. Eating a variety of vegetables and fruits gives you greater flexibility, more choices and additional antioxidants.

The carbohydrate group contains vegetables, fruits, grains, beans and lentils. Vegetables are your best carbohydrate choice for health and healing. Vegetables such as broccoli, cauliflower, greens, bell peppers, lettuce, cabbage, cucumbers and tomatoes are high in fiber, vitamins and minerals. Higher carb choices such as breads, pastas, grains and fruits should be limited.

Benefits of real carbohydrates

Choose a variety of real carbs (fruits and vegetables) instead of man-made, processed carbs. Real carbs, especially vegetables, are key to:

- Balanced blood sugar
- Better metabolism
- Weight loss
- Reduced cravings
- Strong immune function
- Improved digestion

Vegetables (1-3 c. per meal or snack)

- Asparagus
- Bell peppers
- Broccoli
- Brussels sprouts
- Cabbage
- Cauliflower
- Celery
- Cucumber
- Eggplant
- Green beans
- Kale
- Mushrooms
- Salad greens
- Snow peas
- Spinach
- Sugar snap peas
- Summer squash
- Tomatoes
- Water chestnuts
- Zucchini

Vegetables to limit (½ c. per meal or snack)

- Beets
- Carrots
- Corn
- Onions
- Parsnips
- Peas
- Sweet potato
- Yam
- Turnips
- White potato
- Winter squash

Fruits (½ c. per meal or snack)

- Apple
- Banana
- Blackberries
- Blueberries
- Cherries
- Grapefruit
- Grapes
- Kiwi
- Mango
- Melon
- Nectarine
- Orange
- Peach
- Pear
- Pineapple
- Plum
- Strawberries
- Raspberries

Grains, Beans & Lentils (½ c. per meal or snack)

- Beans
- Brown rice
- Lentils
- Millet
- Oats
- Quinoa
- Ryvita® crackers
- Split peas
- Wasa® Lite Rye crackers
- Wild rice

Grains to limit (1 serving per day)

- Bread
- English muffin
- Pita bread
- Rye bread
- Tortilla
- White rice
- Whole grain crackers

Protein

Your body needs protein for energy, tissue repair, blood sugar balance and immune function. Some people may need more protein per day depending on their physical demands, immune function and stress levels. Including protein in a meal can raise your metabolism by as much as thirty percent for up to three to four hours. What a great way for someone looking to lose weight to boost metabolism! By eating small amounts of protein throughout the day, you will keep your metabolism and energy high, provide a sense of well-being and support your immune system.

Benefits of real protein

By eating 2-4 ounces of animal protein at every meal and snack, you will support:

- Metabolism
- Energy
- Immune function
- Focus
- Moods

Fat

Nutritional Weight & Wellness believes that the majority of people benefit from a combination of saturated, monounsaturated and polyunsaturated fats, all of which are necessary for optimal cell health. Pay more attention to the type of fats you are eating than to the amount of fat. For healthy cell membranes, restrict your intake of refined oils and avoid all foods containing partially hydrogenated or hydrogenated fats.

Benefits of real fat

By eating 1-2 tablespoons of beneficial fats per meal or snack, you will support:

- Metabolism
- Cardiovascular system
- Mental and emotional health
- Hormonal balance
- Skin, nails, and hair
- Balanced blood sugar

Protein (4-6 oz. per meal, 2 oz. per snack)

- Beef
- Buffalo
- Chicken
- Eggs
- Fish
- Lamb
- Pork
- Seafood
- Turkey
- Veal
- Venison
- Whey protein

Proteins to limit to one serving per day

- Cottage cheese
- Hard and soft cheeses
- Ricotta cheese
- Soy
- Yogurt

Fats (1-2 Tbsp. per meal or snack)

- Avocado (½)
- Butter
- Coconut oil
- Cream
- Cream cheese
- Mayonnaise
- Nut butters
- Nuts (¼ c.)
- Olive oil
- Olives (10)
- Seeds
- Sesame oil

Food Sensitivities

Are you sensitive to gluten, dairy or soy? A growing number of people are discovering that food sensitivities or intolerances cause a range of health issues from digestive problems to headaches to inflammation. For this reason, the Weight & Wellness Way includes recipes that address common food sensitivities of grain, dairy, soy and peanuts.

- Dairy sensitivities and lactose intolerance to milk, cheese and yogurt cause problems for a number of people.
- Grain sensitivities, especially to gluten grains such as wheat, barley, rye, oats, spelt and kamut, affect large numbers of people. In the most severe cases, people are diagnosed with celiac disease. In milder cases, grain sensitivities show up as bloating, constipation or diarrhea.
- Soy products, including soy burgers, bars and protein drinks, are difficult for many people to digest. Even soy milk can cause bloating, gas and indigestion.
- Peanut allergies have become so prevalent that we substitute almonds, pecans or walnuts in recipes that call for nuts.

Gluten sensitivity and eating gluten free

Thirty percent of people are gluten sensitive. If you experience pain or inflammation, you may feel better following an eating plan with recipes that are primarily gluten free. We have included many gluten free recipes that use wild rice (which is a grass, not a grain). For most people, wild rice does not cause the inflammation response that pasta or gluten products can create. Many Nutritional Weight & Wellness clients experience less inflammation, better immune function and blood sugar balance, along with weight loss when they eat gluten free.

What is gluten?

Things that make you go "mmm"....croissants, lasagna, quesadilla and chocolate chip cookies. What do all of these tempting foods have in common? Gluten. What is gluten? It is a protein found in grains that adds "mouth feel" and a sticky consistency to breads and other foods that many people find irresistible. Unfortunately, if you, like many other Americans, have an allergy or sensitivity to this grain protein, you may have trouble digesting bread, crackers, pasta, baked goods and many other processed foods.

If you have any of the following symptoms, you may be gluten intolerant:

- Chronic aches/pains
- Intestinal problems (bloating, constipation, diarrhea)
- Mental disorders (attention deficit disorder, schizophrenia, anxiety and depression)
- Fatigue
- Food cravings
- Slow metabolism

The Weight & Wellness Way will enable you to enjoy many of your favorite recipes without the adverse effects that gluten can cause. Some recipes are naturally gluten free, while others offer simple substitutions. You can also apply the substitution principles in this cookbook to your own recipes.

Foods with gluten

- Grains (wheat, oats, rye, barley, spelt and kamut)
- Soy sauce, teriyaki sauce and most barbeque sauces
- Many salad dressings
- Many candies (licorice, malt balls, Kit Kat®, Twix®, Milky Way®)

- Beer
- Most thickened sauces (such as alfredo) and gravies
- Most processed entrées, meats, soups, cheeses and frozen meals

Be aware that many processed snacks include gluten in the form of spices.

Foods that are gluten free

- All vegetables and fruits
- Rice (white, brown, wild)
- Quinoa
- Yogurt, milk, cream, cheese
- Nuts, seeds
- Olives
- Oil and butter

If you suspect that you have gluten intolerance, follow our gluten free plan and recipes for at least three to four weeks. For additional help, consult a licensed nutritionist with experience in gluten free diets.

A miniscule amount of gluten is enough to affect some people—even the residues or crumbs that may contaminate an otherwise grain free meal at a restaurant. For this reason, most people find that the most effective way to completely eliminate gluten is to prepare and eat food from their own kitchens. To make this process easier, we have provided simple, gluten free versions of all of our recipes.

Living without gluten

Eliminating foods containing gluten such as bread, pizza, beer, pasta, crackers, cookies, cakes and more can sound like a daunting task. But if you keep it simple by eating real foods, you will find gluten free shopping and cooking does not have to be complicated.

Beware that if you go gluten free to cure what ails you and end up turning mainly to the many processed gluten free products now on the market, you likely will not feel your best. Most gluten free products are highly processed and contain more sugar and fat to simulate the texture and "mouth feel" that gluten brings to foods like bread and crackers.

Try some of these real food ideas to go gluten free the healthy way:

- Breakfast: Organic eggs scrambled in olive oil served with steamed broccoli and ½ c. strawberries.
- Lunch: Easy Salmon Salad (p. 119) served on a bed of greens.
- Dinner: Grilled sirloin steaks served with Sweet Potato Wedges (p. 155) and a side salad topped with olive oil and balsamic vinegar.
- Snacks: A gluten-free meatball, 10 grapes and 8 walnut halves OR 2 ounces of nitrate-free deli meat spread with cream cheese (rolled up) and served with ½ c. raw carrots.

Focus on the positives!

If you are one of the millions of people who are deciding to eat gluten free, it's natural to focus on what you cannot eat...at first. But remember, there are many more foods you can eat than those you cannot. Sweet potatoes, a delicious peach, a rib eye steak hot off the grill, roasted chicken, some good dark chocolate—focus on all of these scrumptious foods and more that you can eat. Believe me, you will not go hungry and in the end, you will see many improvements in your health.

Dairy sensitivity

Dairy products, including milk, cheese and yogurt, cause problems for a number of people. Approximately 70 percent of the world's population is lactose intolerant, which makes it the norm not the exception. Lactose is the carbohydrate or sugar found in milk, including breast milk. As infants, our digestive tracts have the enzyme lactase which breaks down and helps digest the lactose. However, as we age our bodies lose the ability to produce lactase, and we can become lactose intolerant. Symptoms of lactose intolerance include bloating, gas, and diarrhea. These symptoms usually begin 30 minutes to two hours after consuming lactose in milk, ice cream, yogurt, cottage cheese, and pudding.

Many people also have a sensitivity to the casein protein in dairy products. Cheese is a concentrated source of casein because during the cheese-making process, casein thickens and congeals while the whey drains away. Casein molecules are large and can cause inflammation in the gut, as well as throughout the body. Symptoms of casein sensitivity include diarrhea, bloating, abdominal cramps, constipation, joint pain, fatigue, mood disorders, dandruff, eczema or dermatitis, sinus congestion, rosacea, and weight gain.

If you think you may be sensitive to dairy products, try removing milk, yogurt, sour cream, cheese, cottage cheese, pudding, and cream cheese from your diet for six weeks and see how you feel. At Nutritional Weight & Wellness, we have found that most clients can tolerate heavy cream, butter, and ghee during this time, but some people do not. After six weeks, reintroduce these foods for a day or two and notice if those old symptoms return. It shouldn't take long for your body to give you the answer. Some people find they are able to still eat small amounts of these foods on occasion, while others decide it is best to avoid them completely. Listen to your body and decide what is right for you.

Food Additives to Avoid

Everywhere we look, we are constantly bombarded with foods containing artificial sweeteners, such as ice cream, flavored water, cereal, crackers, and teas. Artificial sweeteners are hiding in many processed products. Unfortunately, chemical sweeteners get approved for human consumption before we really know the effects on the body.

Aspartame, found in the blue Equal® packets, is 200 times sweeter than sugar and can cause symptoms such as fatigue, headaches, diarrhea, insomnia, depression, and memory problems. Aspartame is commonly used to sweeten diet soda and is often advertised as being a better choice than regular soda because it contains no calories. Interestingly, a study in the *American Journal of Clinical Nutrition* from the University of Minnesota found a positive association with diet soda consumption and weight gain.

Splenda®, or sucralose, found in the yellow packets, is the newest artificial sweetener. It is 600 times sweeter than sugar and can be found in over 4,000 different food and beverage products. Splenda is advertised as being a "better" sweetener because it is made from sugar, but the process requires adding chlorine to the sugar in order to change its chemical structure. This means that the body is unable to metabolize Splenda in the same way as sugar. A range of symptoms such as skin reactions, joint pain, sinus problems, and heart palpitations have already been connected to Splenda intake. In a study from the *Journal of Toxicology and Environmental Health*, Splenda was found to significantly decrease bifidobacteria in animals' intestinal tracts. We need beneficial bifidobacteria in the intestinal tract to help break down and digest food, absorb nutrients, and eliminate waste. Who would guess that drinking a diet soda may actually reduce good gut bacteria? Another study on Splenda found that it reduced the size of the thymus gland, which is critical for healthy immune function.

Avoid aspartame, sucralose, and saccharin. These have all been linked to many negative side effects.

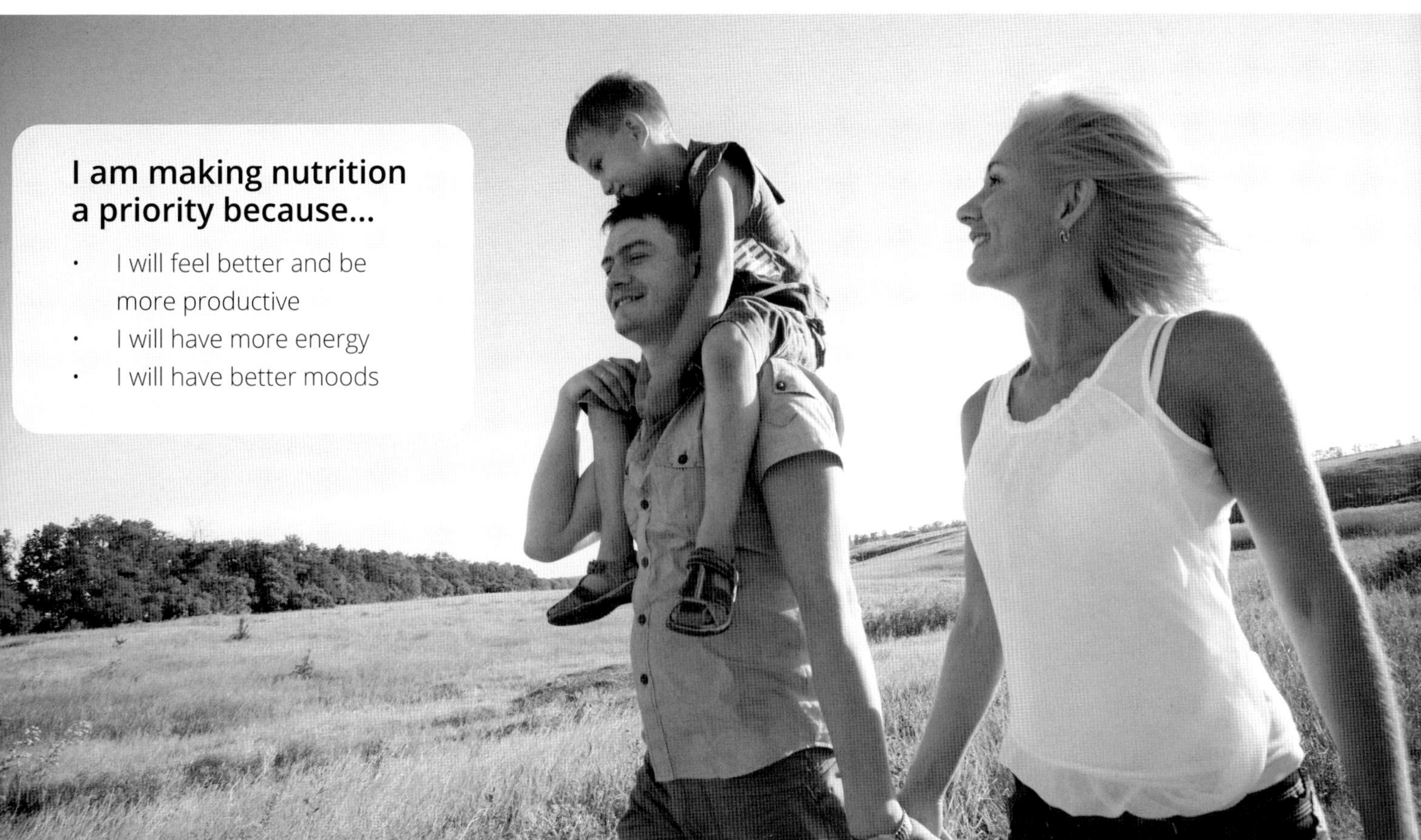
I am making nutrition a priority because...
• I will feel better and be more productive
• I will have more energy
• I will have better moods

Drink Up: The Benefits of Water

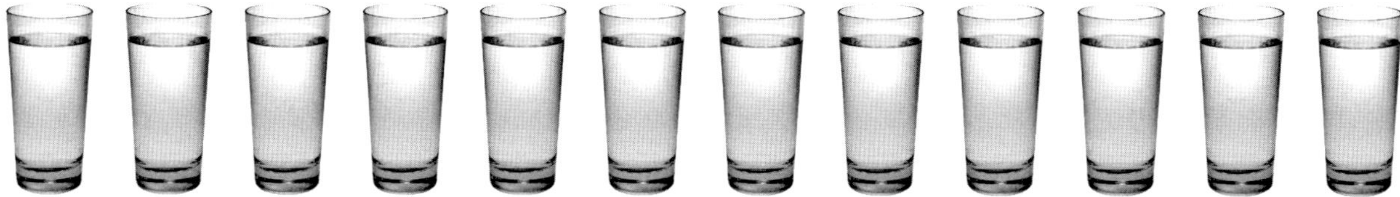

1. The kidneys cannot function properly without enough water

When the kidneys are not functioning properly, the liver must pitch in to help. When the liver is called upon to do some of the kidneys' work, the liver cannot do its job of metabolizing fat efficiently. Therefore, less fat is metabolized, leaving more of it stored in the body as excess weight.

2. Water is key to metabolizing fat

Sufficient water consumption is necessary for the kidneys to function properly, which allows the liver to metabolize fat for energy. Excess weight is burned as energy, resulting in weight loss.

3. Drinking water is essential to weight loss

Overweight people need more water than thin people in order to metabolize stored fat. Adequate water consumption helps to detox the waste from metabolized fat.

4. Water suppresses the appetite naturally

Drinking water throughout the day helps to maintain a normal appetite. At times, hunger may be a sign of dehydration.

5. Water helps relieve constipation

A common symptom of not drinking enough water is constipation. To maintain normal bowel function, drink plenty of water.

6. Water keeps skin supple and youthful

Dehydration in the body leads to skin cells that appear saggy and dry. Drinking sufficient water hydrates tissues throughout the body to prevent wrinkles and dry, rough skin.

Water

Drink 8-10 glasses (8 oz.) of water per day. Avoid soda. Drinking water is critical for:

- Metabolism
- Weight loss
- Skin, nails, and hair
- Energy
- Organ function

Beverages to limit

- Tea (up to 3 c.)
- Coffee (up to 2 c.)
- Milk (up to 1 c.)
- Mineral water (12 oz.)

Beverages to avoid

- Soda – regular and diet
- Juice
- Energy drinks
- Soy milk
- Sweet teas

Keeping Your Blood Sugar Balanced the Weight & Wellness Way

First of all, blood sugar or glucose is one of the substances that the brain and body use for energy, along with the amino acids found in protein and the fatty acids that come from fat. To some extent, every cell relies on glucose. The brain and nervous system need glucose for fuel. The concentration of glucose in your blood stream is called the blood sugar level. The healthy blood sugar range is between 70 and 95 milligrams. Recent research shows that when people keep their blood sugar below 95, they maintain healthy cells and do not age as quickly.

Blood sugar balance is crucial for long-term health. For most people, obesity, diabetes and heart disease result from high blood sugar levels. Over time, high blood sugar levels will damage each and every cell in your body.

When blood sugar levels are too high:

- Inflammation occurs throughout the body, including the lungs, joints and brain.
- The effectiveness of the immune system decreases up to 50 percent for several hours.
- Hormonal balance becomes disrupted and you experience more PMS (cramps, fluid retention) or menopause symptoms (hot flashes).
- Bones weaken, leading to osteoporosis.
- High blood pressure and high cholesterol can be other consequences.
- Insomnia can set in.

When blood sugar levels drop below 70, the brain sends a message to the body that it needs glucose. The body then craves sweets, and you reach for the candy dish.

The Weight & Wellness Way to balanced blood sugar

Many of us are not conscious of our own blood sugar level. After eating highly processed carbohydrates, such as bagels, your blood sugar level goes sky high. The hormone, insulin, is released to rebalance the glucose in the blood stream. At that point, the cells receive too much insulin, dropping the blood sugar too low, and you crave sugar, continuing the vicious cycle. When you skip meals, you also set yourself up for low blood sugar and cravings.

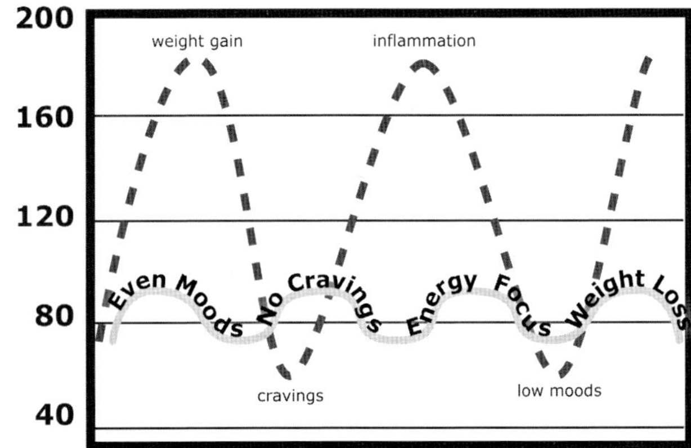

Balanced blood sugar = good health

What is the solution? Follow the Weight & Wellness Way to balance blood sugar by eating five to six small meals containing protein, carbohydrates and healthy fat.

- Vegetable carbohydrates, low in sugar content and high in fiber, support blood sugar balance more effectively than processed carbohydrates.
- Protein stimulates the release of glucagon, a hormone that supports blood sugar balance and metabolism.
- Adding good fat to meals and snacks helps stabilize blood sugar, slows the rate at which carbohydrates break down, keeps you full longer and reduces cravings.

The Weight & Wellness Way to Control Cravings

Does this program work for compulsive eaters?

Yes, the Weight & Wellness Way strategy for controlling cravings is built on the four major biochemical factors that lead to cravings, overeating or compulsive eating.

1. Blood sugar balance: When your blood sugar drops too low, you crave sugar. People who follow low fat diets or who overeat carbohydrates have more difficulty managing their blood sugar. If you don't eat a balance of protein, carbohydrates and fats at each meal and snack, you set yourself up for cravings and overeating.
2. Poor intestinal health: Cravings and compulsive eating often come from poor intestinal health which may occur after the use of antibiotics or anti-inflammatory drugs. Eating foods that contain bifidobacteria (yogurt, sauerkraut and kefir) may help reduce these cravings, but most people need to take a bifidobacteria supplement.
3. Insufficient neurotransmitters: Consuming insufficient protein to produce the "feel good" chemicals that help regulate our eating can result in low neurotransmitter levels. People who are deficient in serotonin or other "feel good" brain chemicals often experience low moods and strong cravings for sugar and carbohydrates. The Weight & Wellness plan recommends eating 12-14 ounces of animal protein per day for the production of these "feel good" brain chemicals. An easy way to get more protein is to whip up a protein shake every day. Try our easy shake recipe (p. 40) in the Breakfast section of this book.
4. Mineral and vitamin deficiencies: Many people experience out-of-control compulsive eating when they are deficient in key minerals such as zinc and certain vitamins, such as vitamin D. Working one-on-one with a nutritionist is helpful to identify and correct vitamin and mineral deficiencies.

Robert's success story–discovering how to break the addictive process

The moment I eat food high in carbohydrates, especially sugar or flour, the pattern of cravings and increased hunger takes over. My behavior gets erratic; I experience obsessive thoughts about donuts, ice cream, cookies and cake. The sight of those foods proves too strong a trigger and I cave in. That is the compulsive side of my disease.

I have no control over food. This notion is a bit tricky for me. It is not a black and white issue. I have found that when I abstain from processed sugar, flour and grain and foods containing those ingredients, I break the addictive process. That means that my hunger returns to normal (as manageable). It also means that cravings subside to a manageable level. This is due to the stabilization of my blood sugar.

Tips For Eating The Weight and Wellness Way

1. **Be realistic** when setting goals. Change at a rate that is comfortable for you.

2. **Be consistent**. Make changes that will improve your health and practice those changes until they become a permanent part of your lifestyle.

3. **Plan ahead**. Have the right foods on hand (especially protein) to avoid high-risk situations—being too hungry, overly stressed or emotionally charged—that can steer you off course.

4. **Surround yourself** with people who support your desire to change.

5. **Exercise regularly** if you are not already doing so. Exercise helps manage your moods, build your immune system and increase your energy.

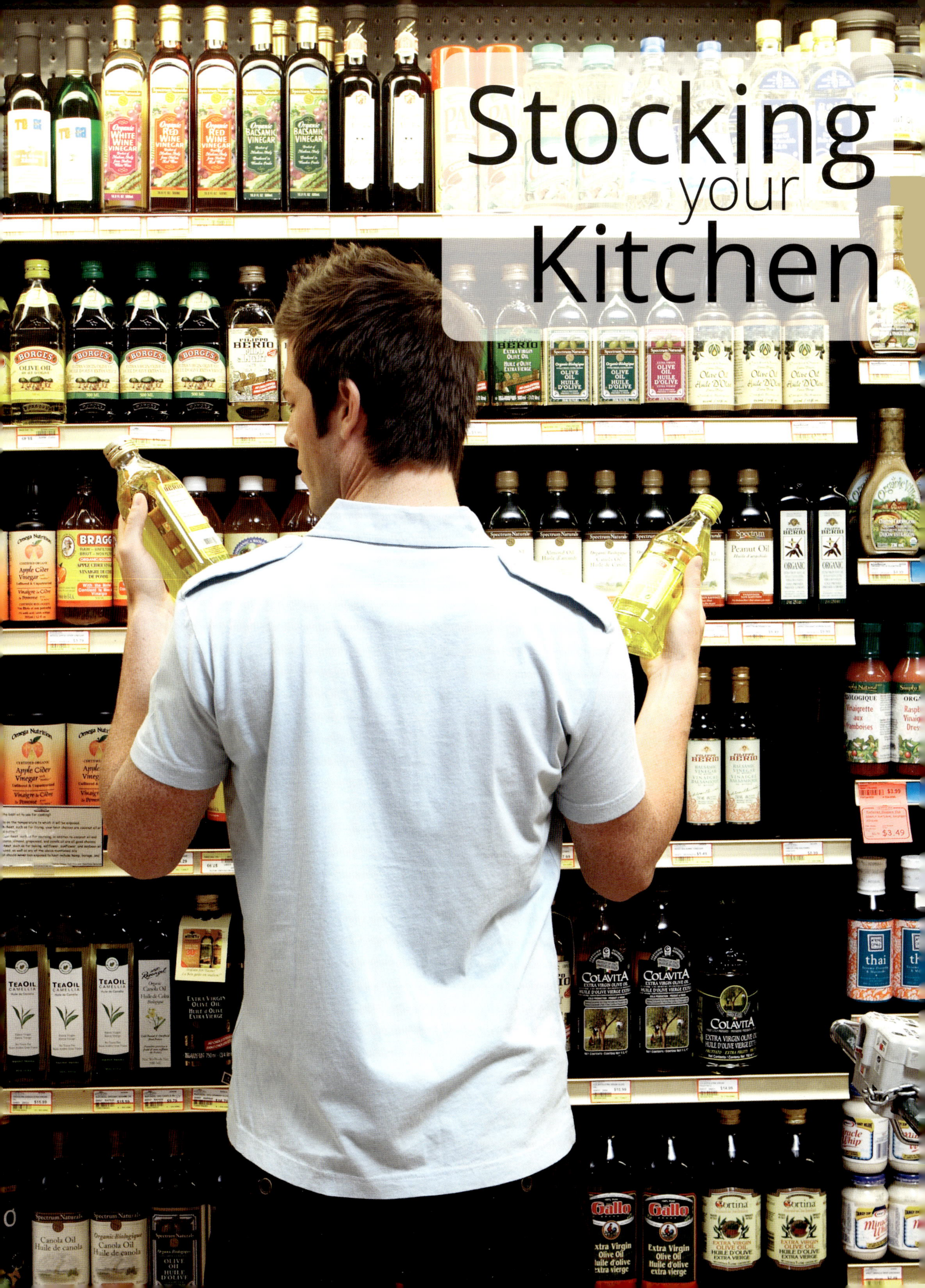

Stocking your Kitchen

Stocking Your Kitchen

Shopping Tips

The first steps to cooking healthy meals are knowing how to shop and what foods to stock in your kitchen. The following shopping tips will make building balance meals a breeze. Remember, the goal is to prepare nutritious meals quickly and easily without continuously reinventing the wheel at each meal.

To prepare meals quickly, it helps to buy ingredients in their most usable form. Purchasing chicken or turkey that is skinless and boneless or precooked deli meats from a natural foods store or co-op saves you time. Cheese can be pre-sliced or shredded. Salad greens can be prewashed, sliced or bagged. Fresh fruit may also be cubed and packaged. Stock up on your favorite fruits and vegetables, both fresh and frozen.

Visit the farmers market for a wide selection of fresh, seasonal produce, meat and eggs. Buying directly from farmers connects us to the earth and to the people who provide our food. Shopping at the farmers market is a fun family field trip.

Protein

Red meat

Buy grass-fed or organic meat as often as your budget allows. Organic meat is free of antibiotics, growth hormones and toxic chemicals that interfere with healing.

Poultry

We encourage you to purchase organic or free-range poultry when possible. You will be amazed at the difference in taste between a roasted organic or free-range chicken and one from the meat counter at a conventional grocery store. Baby Boomers comment that organic chicken reminds them of the chicken from grandma's farm. Also, look for frozen organic chicken or turkey sausage or brats without nitrates or chemical additives. They are a healthy way to add protein at breakfast.

Fish

Whether fresh, frozen or canned in water, fish is an excellent source of protein. Salmon, sardines and mackerel are rich in healthy Omega-3 fatty acids. All fish cooks quickly, and canned fish, such as salmon and sardines, come ready to eat for convenient snacking. Safeguard against eating fish with high levels of pollutants, such as PCBs and mercury by consulting the United States Environmental Protection Agency.

Eggs

Certainly, eggs do not deserve the reputation that they have acquired during the past decades of cholesterol bashing and fat-free merchandising. Eggs are one of the most readily available sources of protein that we can consume. They have long

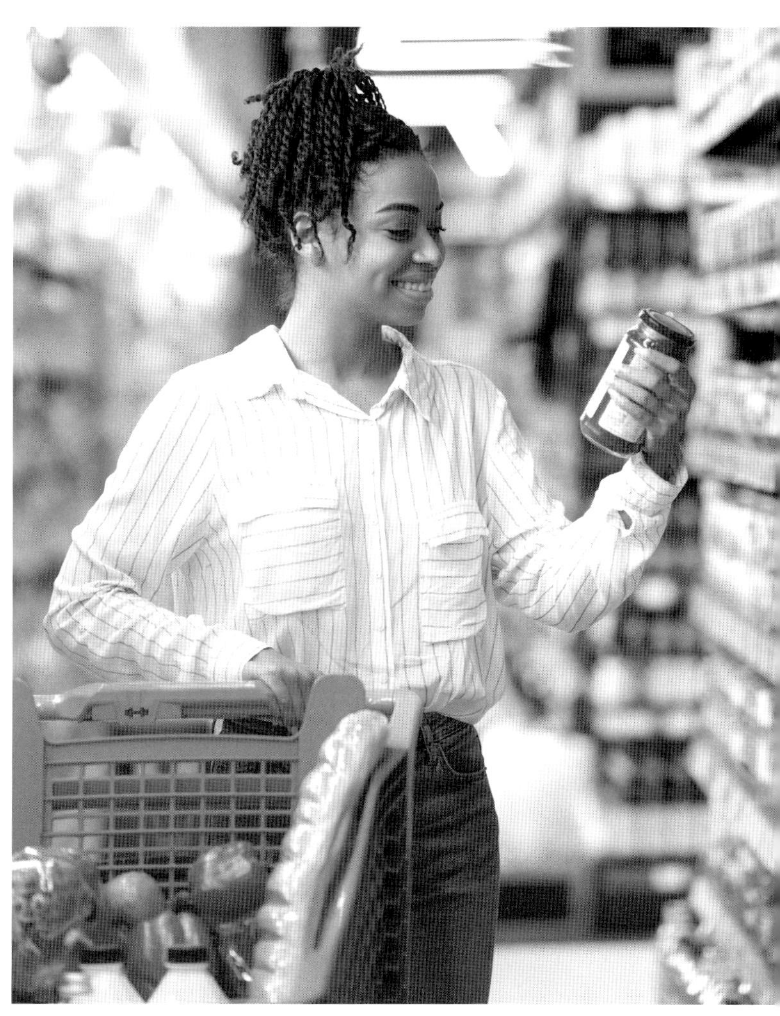

been regarded as the standard against which all other protein is judged.

Cholesterol is necessary for hormone function and only needs to be avoided if it has been oxidized. This oxidized cholesterol is found in foods that have been processed: powdered milk, powdered eggs and processed baked goods (muffins, cakes, donuts, etc.).

Yolks from grocery store eggs can retain toxic residues from the growth hormones, pesticides and antibiotics fed to chickens that are commercially raised. Therefore, we recommend that you buy free-range or organic eggs. Because of what these chickens are fed, the yolks of their eggs have less saturated fat and more of the essential Omega-3 fats. You will be surprised at the dramatic flavor differences in organic eggs.

Other meats

You may be surprised by the variety of meats available at your supermarket today. Try bison, ostrich, rabbit or venison. You may have lean, wild game in the freezer if you have a hunter in the family.

If you eat pork, we recommend pastured (free-range) pork because of the high level of antibiotics fed to pigs in feedlots and large, commercial operations.

From the Dairy Case

Milk and yogurt

Current research supports the importance of saturated fats for health; therefore, Nutritional Weight & Wellness recommends organic, full-fat dairy products. You can find organic yogurt with active cultures at neighborhood co-ops or grocery stores with organic and whole foods sections.

Cottage cheese

Buy organic cottage cheese whenever possible. If you cannot find organic cottage cheese, we recommend one or two percent because of the added hormones and antibiotics in conventional cottage cheese.

Cheese

Avoid fat-free cheeses. They are loaded with sodium, sugar and artificial flavor enhancers. Use real cheese, in moderation, to add flavor to a meal. We recommend organic or imported cheeses that are hormone and antibiotic free. For people who are dairy sensitive, goat cheese is a good alternative. Avoid soy cheeses as they contain too many additives.

Vegetarian Protein

Tofu

Made from soybean curds, tofu is an alternative source of protein. Organic tofu is inexpensive, low in chemical toxins and contains essential fatty acids. When eating vegetable protein, balance it with eggs or cheese to form a complete protein.

Soy milk and soy products

We do not recommend using soy milk, but if you do, select a brand that is organic and low in carbohydrates. Most soy burgers, hot dogs and other soy products, such as textured vegetable protein, are highly processed and contain a lot of additives. Many processed soy products also contain refined sugars and preservatives. Another concern today is that most soy products come from genetically modified soybeans, and the health effects of these modifications are unknown.

Beans

Although vegetarians consider beans to be a protein source, beans contain twice as much carbohydrate as they do protein, and the protein in beans is not as usable to the body as the protein found in animal sources. Consider beans and legumes as carbohydrates.

Carbohydrates

Build your carbohydrate choices around vegetables and fruit and you'll come out a winner. For optimal health, we recommend five to nine servings of vegetables per day, emphasizing variety. Fresh and frozen, low and high carb choices, all in balance add to your health. Think color: red, yellow, orange and green. Think fiber.

Vegetables

Choose fresh or frozen vegetables. Visit the salad bar at your supermarket for convenience. Look for cauliflower and broccoli florets, pre-cut vegetables and organic, leafy greens for easy tossing. A bag of mixed vegetables already cleaned and chopped saves time. Fresh greens, such as spinach, are good any time—even for breakfast. Serve greens on the side or in an omelet. Fresh, organic mixed greens are easy to find and are packed with healing nutrients.

The only canned vegetable you should use regularly is a canned tomato product. Reading labels on tomato products (sauces, stewed, chopped or whole) is important because many of these products contain preservatives.

Beans

Beans provide a powerhouse of high fiber carbohydrate and additional protein to your meal. When not using fresh or dried, look for canned, organic beans from the health food section of your grocery. They are the most nutritious choice.

Fruits

Nutritious and economical, fruits provide vitamins, fiber, antioxidants and a range of nutrients important to your health. Many stores carry fresh fruit that has already been cleaned and cut for convenience. Don't rely solely on citrus and apples. Consider melons, kiwi, mangos, papaya, raspberries, etc. for variety. Unsweetened frozen fruits and those canned in their own juices are good staples to have on hand. Avoid fruit juices, which are naturally high in sugar, and eat the whole fruit instead.

Breads and Grains

Bread

If you are choosing bread as your carbohydrate instead of vegetables, then you will want the most nutrient-dense, whole grain bread you can find. The best bread for stable blood sugar is 100 percent whole grain rye. You have to search diligently to find rye bread without added wheat flour. Choose breads that do not contain preservatives, partially hydrogenated oil or sugar. Trust us; you have to check the ingredient list when buying bread. Look for whole grain as the first ingredient.

Crackers

Avoid highly processed crackers containing refined oils. Wasa® and Ryvita® crackers made from whole rye flour are readily available at major grocery store chains. You may discover other whole grain flat bread crackers.

Healthy Fats

At Nutritional Weight & Wellness, we are firm believers in the importance of fats in the diet for health and healing. In the field of nutrition, there has been ongoing controversy about the role of fat in the diet and a lack of appreciation for the value of healthy fats. Misinformation, fueled by advertising campaigns by food manufacturers, has led Americans to replace traditional fat sources, such as butter and coconut oil, with unhealthy fats, such as Crisco®, margarine and soybean oil. Even within the health care professions, a lack of scientific information has led to promotion of unhealthy fats such as margarine and corn oil.

In the past, we have been cautioned about the use of saturated fat. Mary Enig, leading researcher and author of *Know Your Fats*, explains the complementary roles of saturated, monounsaturated and polyunsaturated fats in cell health. The Weight & Wellness Way is based on scientific information, and research recommends a balance of saturated, polyunsaturated and monounsaturated fat. Consume healthy fats and oils, not damaged fats (those with hydrogenated or partially hydrogenated oil.)

Beneficial fats

- Nuts (raw)
- Olives and olive oil
- Avocados
- Butter or ghee
- Seeds
- Coconut oil

Shopping for fats

- When possible, use organic sources of fats because toxins, preservatives and additives are stored in fats. Buy organic butter, organic cold-pressed olive oil and organic nuts and seeds.
- Buy raw nuts and roast your own.
- Avoid processed, prepared foods. They are a source of refined, damaged oils.
- Don't buy refined oil, such as corn, soybean or vegetable oil.
- Avoid any nuts and seeds roasted in refined oils, such as cottonseed or soybean oil.

Preservative-Free Ingredients

In addition to choosing natural foods for optimal nutrition, you also want to use preservative-free sweeteners, sauces and marinades. Here are better options to replace artificial sweeteners and commercial soy sauce.

Vegetable glycerine

Derived from coconut, vegetable glycerine is non-toxic and easy to digest. Even though the body metabolizes it like a carbohydrate, vegetable glycerine does not disrupt blood sugar levels or cause an insulin response. It makes an excellent sugar substitute for beverages, shakes and baked goods.

Stevia

The naturally sweet herb stevia grows in South America and works well for sweetening beverages and in cooking when used in moderation. Because stevia is highly concentrated, a small amount goes a long way.

Pure Maple Syrup

This versatile natural sweetener tastes delicious and does not increase sugar cravings for most people. Make sure you buy 100% pure maple syrup.

Bragg® Liquid Aminos

This natural blend of amino acids makes this soy product an excellent replacement for commercial soy sauce. It does not contain wheat, MSG (monosodium glutamate) or other additives to which people often are sensitive. Substitute Bragg Liquid Aminos in any recipe calling for soy sauce, natural shoyu, tamari or miso. You will find that it adds great flavor to meats, salad dressings and stir-fry dishes.

Organic Broths

Natural food stores and large grocery stores offer a variety of organic and free-range chicken, beef and vegetable broths. These flavorful broths are far healthier and often lower in sodium than the commercially available brands that rely on MSG, preservatives and other flavor enhancers. Because organic broths do not contain preservatives, once opened they need to be refrigerated and used within seven days.

Dangers of Cooking with Aluminum Foil

Cooking in aluminum foil is not safe according to research published in the International Journal of Electrochemical Science, May 2012.

Minimal exposure of aluminum (60mg/day) to our bodies is not a problem, but meals cooked in the oven wrapped in aluminum foil were found to contain 400 mg of aluminum. The amount of aluminum leaching into food was greater when it was cooked at higher temperatures with vinegar and added spices. Foil is not safe for cooking and is not suitable for use with vegetables such as tomatoes, citrus juices and many spices.

Health risk of excess aluminum:

- Aluminum salts can be absorbed by the gut and become concentrated in various human tissues including the bone, parathyroid and brain.
- High concentrations of aluminum have been detected in patients with Alzheimer's disease.
- High aluminum intakes may also be harmful to some patients with bone and renal impairments because aluminum competes with calcium, thus weakening the bones.

What's a better choice?

For oven cooking, we recommend using parchment paper. It's a safe and versatile alternative to aluminum foil.

For grilling, we recommend using a grill basket instead of aluminum foil.

Cooking with Parchment

You can buy parchment bags or make your own with parchment paper. Parchment bags or parchment paper can be purchased online or found at many grocery stores.

Try these recipes:

- Asian Beef and Vegetable Meal-in-a-Bag (p. 47)
- Chicken and Vegetable Meal-in-a-Bag (p. 64)
- Turkey and Vegetable Meal-in-a-Bag (p. 88)

The Weight & Wellness Way to a Healthy Heart

What will happen to my cholesterol when eating this way?

If you are concerned about your cholesterol numbers, following this eating plan usually raises HDL (good cholesterol) and lowers LDL (bad cholesterol). Seventy to eighty percent of cholesterol is made in your body—only twenty to thirty percent comes from dietary sources.

Eggs, animal protein and healthy saturated fats are not the culprits behind elevated cholesterol levels. Although in the past saturated fats have been identified as the source of cholesterol problems, the true culprits are the bad fats and refined oils found in margarine and many processed foods. Damaged fats represent one of the single greatest dietary threats to our overall health, particularly to our blood vessels. If you have high cholesterol, Nutritional Weight & Wellness strongly recommends avoiding bad fats. Do not buy products that contain hydrogenated or partially hydrogenated fats or oils. Most people who follow a balanced eating plan that eliminates bad fats and reduces sugar and processed carbohydrates have healthy cholesterol numbers.

Becky's success story–better cholesterol numbers and more energy

I have struggled with high cholesterol for over 20 years. When I went to Nutritional Weight & Wellness, my total cholesterol was 264 and my triglycerides hit 427. After just seven months of healthy, balanced eating and nutritional supplements, my total cholesterol dropped from 264 to 210 and my triglycerides went from 427 to 222! I did this without increasing my exercise or making any other changes.

What amazes me even more is that my cholesterol improved while I was eating eggs fried in butter and having cottage cheese with nuts, even though my doctor told me to cut back on fat, especially saturated fat.

Overall, I feel more aware of my body. For the first time, I make a connection between what I eat and how I feel. Eating eggs for breakfast has made a big difference in my energy. (I used to fall asleep after eating pancakes and syrup.) I even found it really easy to eat this way when I went on a cruise.

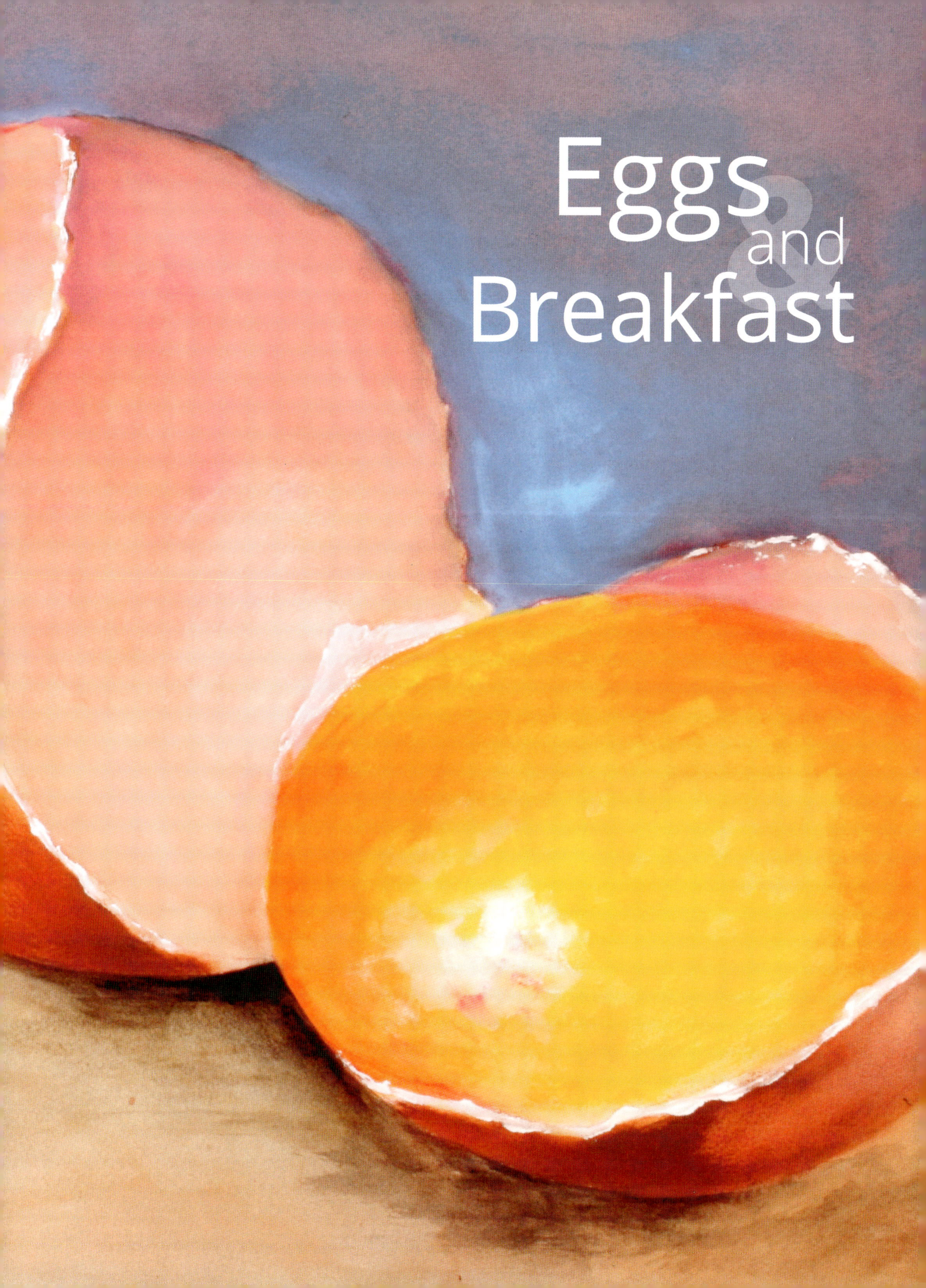
Eggs
&
and
Breakfast

Blueberry Muffins

2 ½ c. almond flour
½ c. whey protein powder
1½ tsp. cinnamon
1 tsp. baking soda
½ tsp. salt

Preheat oven to 350º.

Mix in a large bowl, do not overmix.

⅓ c. coconut oil - melted
4 eggs
¼ c. vegetable glycerine or maple syrup
1 tsp. vanilla

Mix in a blender or with a whisk until smooth.

Stir into dry ingredients.

1½ c. blueberries (or chopped apples)

Gently fold in.

Grease muffin tins with coconut oil. Fill muffin tins 2/3 full.

Bake for 15-20 minutes.

Makes 12 muffins.

Serves 12

This is a balanced snack.

To make gluten free:
This recipe is gluten free

To make dairy free:
Use egg white protein powder or paleo protein powder

Fiction	Fact
Cereal bars are good for you because they have fruit and fiber.	Most cereal bars contain 8 tsp. of sugar, usually high fructose corn syrup. Cereal bars often have hydrogenated or partially hydrogenated oils, which are the damaging fats. A healthier snack would be an apple, a handful of almonds and a hard-boiled egg.

Breakfast Hash with Brussels Sprouts

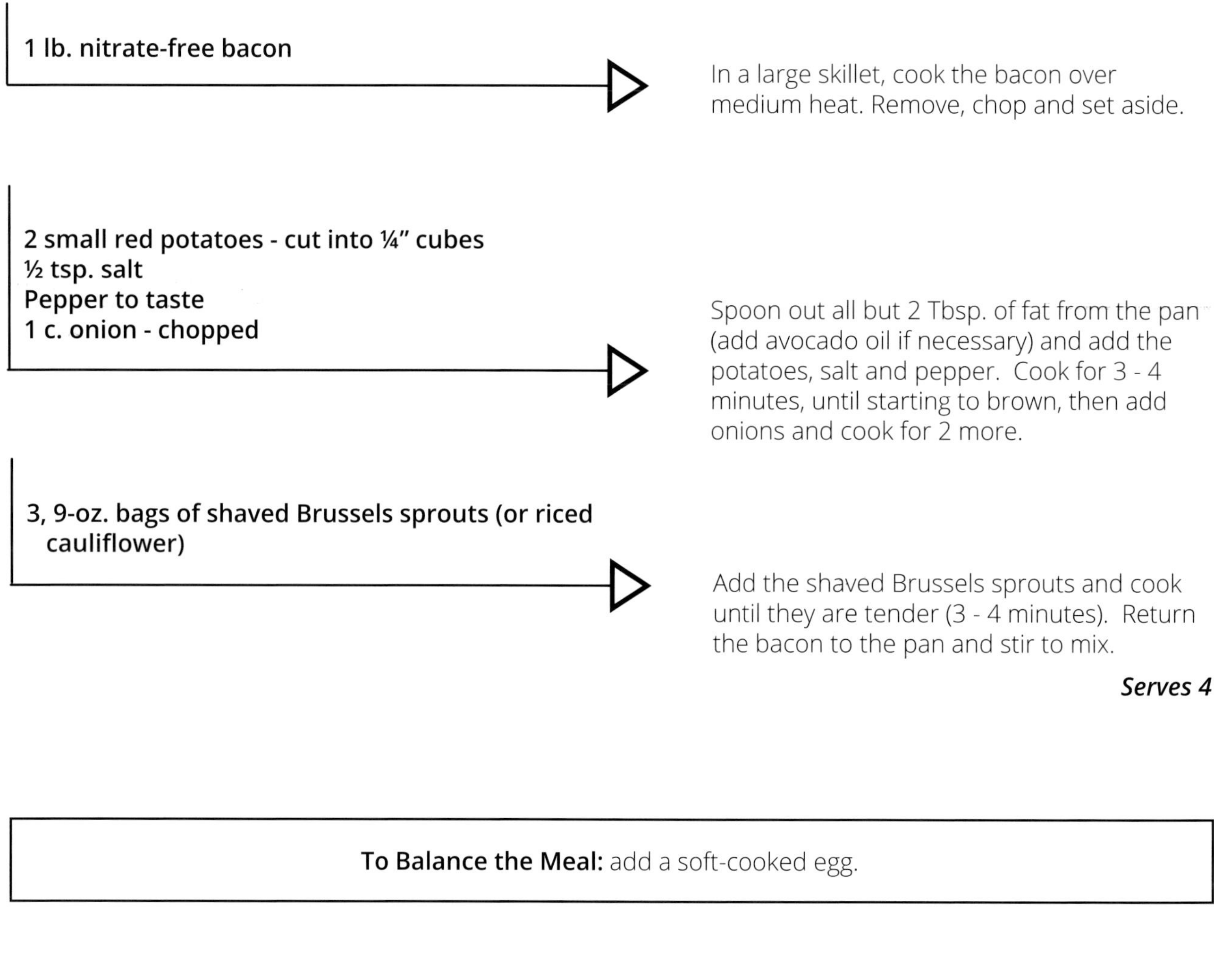

1 lb. nitrate-free bacon

In a large skillet, cook the bacon over medium heat. Remove, chop and set aside.

2 small red potatoes - cut into ¼" cubes
½ tsp. salt
Pepper to taste
1 c. onion - chopped

Spoon out all but 2 Tbsp. of fat from the pan (add avocado oil if necessary) and add the potatoes, salt and pepper. Cook for 3 - 4 minutes, until starting to brown, then add onions and cook for 2 more.

3, 9-oz. bags of shaved Brussels sprouts (or riced cauliflower)

Add the shaved Brussels sprouts and cook until they are tender (3 - 4 minutes). Return the bacon to the pan and stir to mix.

Serves 4

To Balance the Meal: add a soft-cooked egg.

To make gluten free:
This dish is gluten free

To make dairy free:
This dish is dairy free

Breakfast Taco

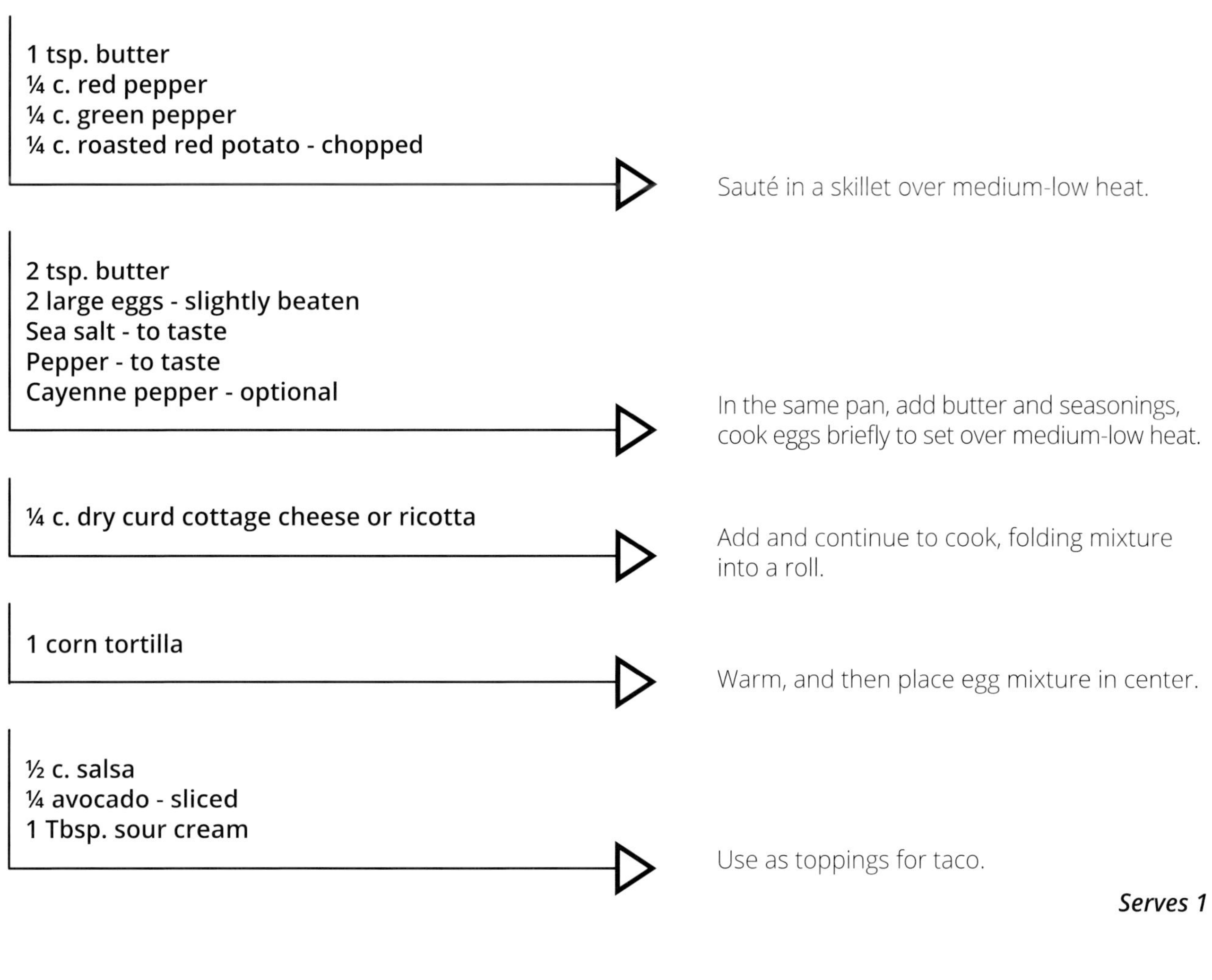

1 tsp. butter
¼ c. red pepper
¼ c. green pepper
¼ c. roasted red potato - chopped

Sauté in a skillet over medium-low heat.

2 tsp. butter
2 large eggs - slightly beaten
Sea salt - to taste
Pepper - to taste
Cayenne pepper - optional

In the same pan, add butter and seasonings, cook eggs briefly to set over medium-low heat.

¼ c. dry curd cottage cheese or ricotta

Add and continue to cook, folding mixture into a roll.

1 corn tortilla

Warm, and then place egg mixture in center.

½ c. salsa
¼ avocado - sliced
1 Tbsp. sour cream

Use as toppings for taco.

Serves 1

To Balance the Meal: this is a balanced meal.

To make gluten free:
Use a gluten free tortilla

To make dairy free:
This meal cannot be made dairy free

Cottage Cheese Apple Pancakes

¾ c. apple (1 large or 2 small apples) - peeled and grated

Peel, core and grate the apple(s) into a mixing bowl.

½ c. small-curd cottage cheese (dry curd or press out the liquid)
2 large eggs
½ tsp. cinnamon
⅛ tsp. nutmeg - optional
1 Tbsp. maple syrup
¼ tsp. salt

Thoroughly mix into the grated apples.

¼ c. almond meal
2 scoops whey protein powder
1 tsp. baking powder

Sprinkle into mixture and stir well.

1 Tbsp. coconut oil
(butter or olive oil may be substituted)
2 tsp. sour cream or crème fraîche

Oil or butter a heavy griddle or skillet and place it on medium heat.

For each pancake, ladle ¼ c. of batter onto the hot griddle.

When bubbles form on the top, the bottoms are browned, flip the pancakes and brown on the other side.

Serve immediately, with sour cream or crème fraîche.

Serves 2

To Balance the Meal: this is a balanced meal.

To make gluten free:
This meal is gluten free

To make dairy free:
This dish cannot be made dairy free

Deviled Eggs

8 eggs

In a saucepan, bring 6 cups of water to a boil.

Using a spoon, gently place eggs in the water, lower the heat to low simmer for 9 minutes.

Remove from heat and rinse under cold water before peeling.

4 Tbsp. mayonnaise (avocado, safflower, or olive oil)
1 tsp. vinegar
Salt to taste
Dash white pepper
½ tsp. dry mustard or 1 tsp. prepared mustard
½ tsp. paprika

Cut hard-boiled eggs in half lengthwise, remove yolks and mash with remaining ingredients.

Refill egg whites, sprinkle with paprika and refrigerate or serve immediately.

Serves 4

To Balance the Snack: serve with ½ apple or ½ c. berries.

To make gluten free:
This meal is gluten free

To make dairy free:
This meal is dairy free

Egg Bake

12 eggs
¾ c. heavy cream or coconut milk
1 tsp. salt
½ tsp. pepper
2 Tbsp. fresh herbs, chopped

Preheat oven to 350°. Grease a 13″ x 9″ pan with butter or olive oil.

Whisk eggs and cream together in a mixing bowl.

1, 12-oz. package hash browns - thawed

Spread hash browns on bottom of pan.

2 Tbsp. ghee or avocado oil
10 oz. fresh or frozen spinach - thawed

Sauté spinach in butter or olive oil and layer over hash browns.

6 oz. nitrate-free sausage links or patties - cooked, cut up
½ c. shredded cheese (cheddar, pepperjack)

Top the hashbrowns with the diced sausage.

Pour egg mixture over sausage.

Bake 35-45 minutes. Sprinkle shredded cheese over top for last 5 minutes of baking.

Serves 6

To Balance the Meal: serve with ½ c. berries.

To make gluten free:
This is gluten free

To make dairy free:
Replace cream with coconut milk and omit cheese

Fact VS. Fiction

Fiction	Fact
Fat is bad for you. Low-fat food is healthier.	Certainly, some low-fat foods are healthy—vegetables and fruits. When the fat is removed from foods naturally containing fat, such as yogurt, food manufactures add sugar and other chemicals to make it taste good, and in the process, make the food unhealthy.

Fast Frittata

1 Tbsp. avocado oil
2 c. large kale or swiss chard leaves - stems removed and chopped
½ small onion - diced
1 c. mushrooms - chopped

Preheat oven broiler.

Sauté onions and mushrooms over medium heat in a 12" skillet until translucent, then add kale or swiss chard and cook until wilted.

¼ c. heavy cream (use coconut cream for dairy free)
10 eggs
2 Tbsp. dill
1 tsp. salt

Whisk eggs, salt, herbs and cream together and pour over vegetables. Do not stir, let the eggs set over med-low heat, careful not to burn the bottom.

2 oz. chèvre or feta cheese (omit if dairy free)

When you see small bubbles rising to the surface of the egg mixture, top with crumbled cheese and place under the broiler in lower third of oven. Cook for 5 minutes or until the eggs are puffed up and cooked through. Let stand for 5 minutes before slicing.

Serves 2

To Balance the Meal: serve with ½ c. fresh fruit.

To make gluten free:
This is gluten free

To make dairy free:
Use coconut cream instead of heavy cream and omit the cheese

Fiction	Fact
I eat cereal for breakfast, and that is a healthy option with vitamins.	Most of the vitamins and minerals that are added to cereals are poor quality and poorly absorbed. Fruit and vegetable carbohydrates provide the body with highly absorbable forms of vitamins and minerals and just the right amount of fiber. Plus, eating just 1 cup of cereal breaks down to about 14 tsp. of sugar!

Protein Shakes

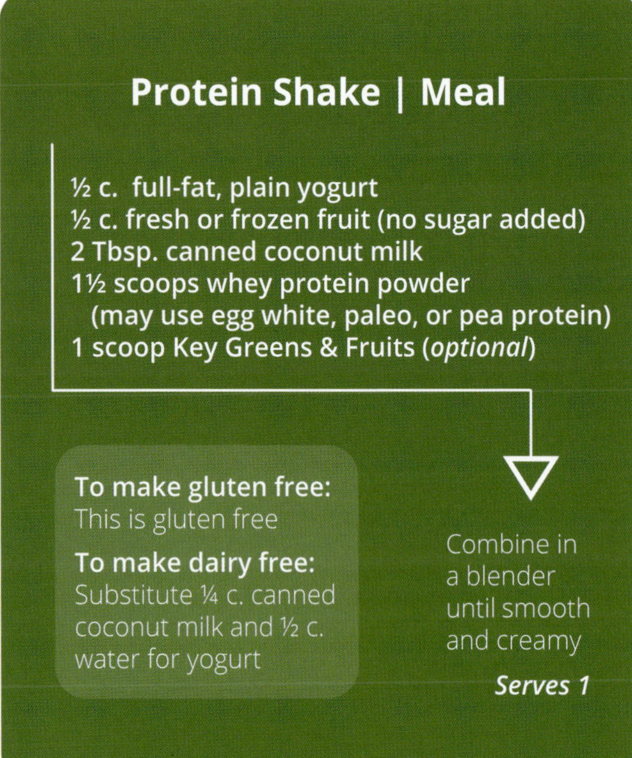

Protein Shake | Meal

½ c. full-fat, plain yogurt
½ c. fresh or frozen fruit (no sugar added)
2 Tbsp. canned coconut milk
1½ scoops whey protein powder
(may use egg white, paleo, or pea protein)
1 scoop Key Greens & Fruits (*optional*)

To make gluten free:
This is gluten free

To make dairy free:
Substitute ¼ c. canned coconut milk and ½ c. water for yogurt

Combine in a blender until smooth and creamy

Serves 1

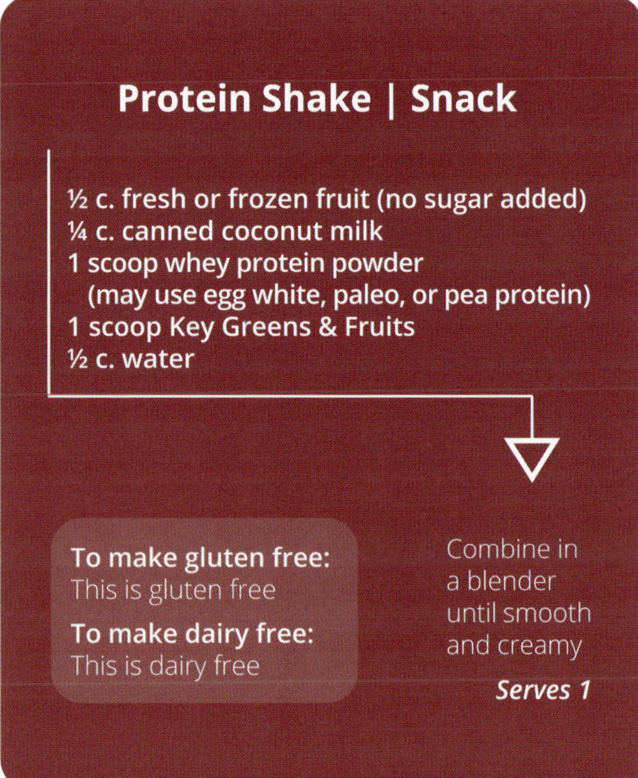

Protein Shake | Snack

½ c. fresh or frozen fruit (no sugar added)
¼ c. canned coconut milk
1 scoop whey protein powder
(may use egg white, paleo, or pea protein)
1 scoop Key Greens & Fruits
½ c. water

To make gluten free:
This is gluten free

To make dairy free:
This is dairy free

Combine in a blender until smooth and creamy

Serves 1

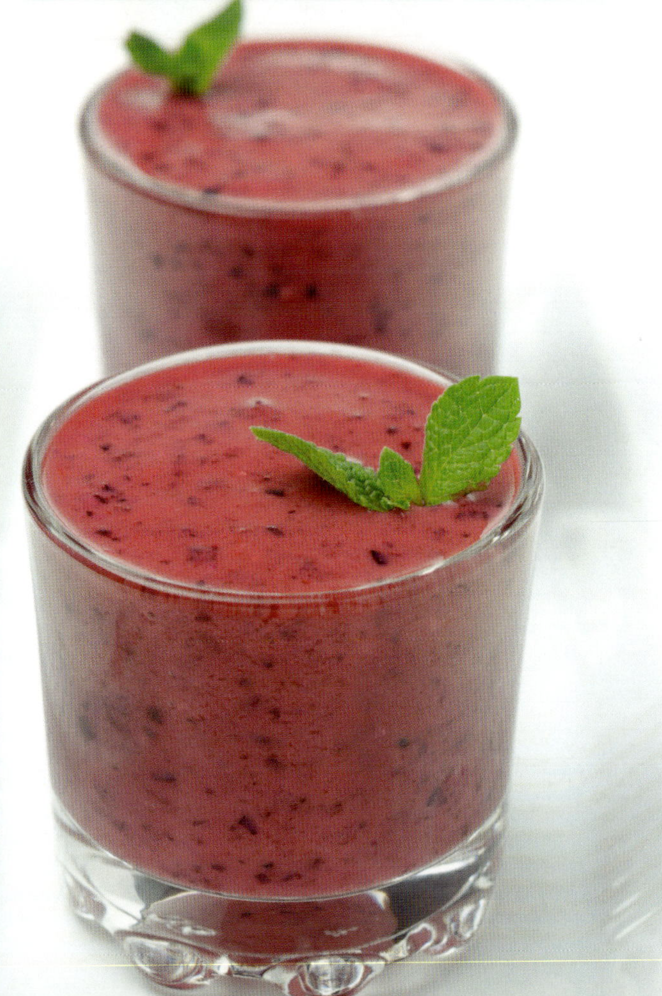

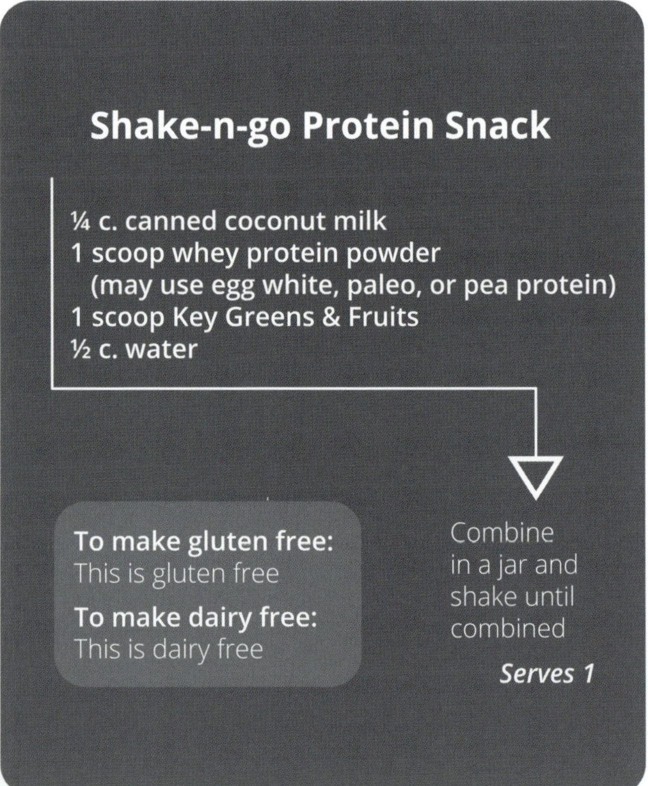

Shake-n-go Protein Snack

¼ c. canned coconut milk
1 scoop whey protein powder
(may use egg white, paleo, or pea protein)
1 scoop Key Greens & Fruits
½ c. water

To make gluten free:
This is gluten free

To make dairy free:
This is dairy free

Combine in a jar and shake until combined

Serves 1

Tofu Scrambler

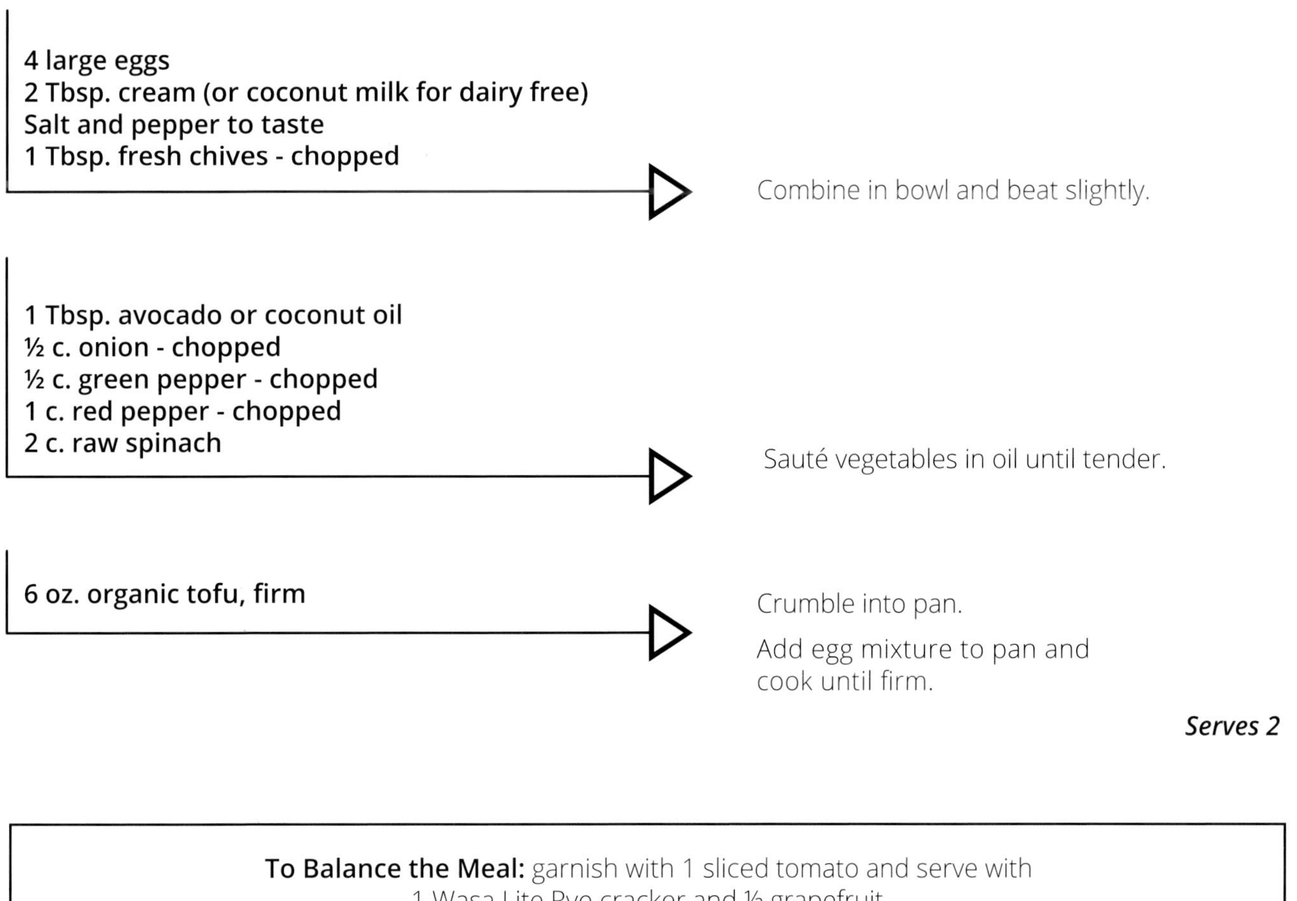

4 large eggs
2 Tbsp. cream (or coconut milk for dairy free)
Salt and pepper to taste
1 Tbsp. fresh chives - chopped

Combine in bowl and beat slightly.

1 Tbsp. avocado or coconut oil
½ c. onion - chopped
½ c. green pepper - chopped
1 c. red pepper - chopped
2 c. raw spinach

Sauté vegetables in oil until tender.

6 oz. organic tofu, firm

Crumble into pan.

Add egg mixture to pan and cook until firm.

Serves 2

To Balance the Meal: garnish with 1 sliced tomato and serve with 1 Wasa Lite Rye cracker and ½ grapefruit.

To make gluten free:
Substitute gluten-free crackers

To make dairy free:
Substitute coconut milk for the cream

Turkey Breakfast Sausages

1 lb. ground turkey
1 tsp. salt
¾ tsp. pepper
1 tsp. dried sage
2 tsp. fennel seed
⅛ tsp. red pepper flakes
2 tsp. avocado or coconut oil

In a bowl, mix spices thoroughly into ground turkey.

Divide evenly into 8 patties.

Heat a sauté pan to medium-high and add avocado oil. Add turkey sausage and cook through, about 3 - 4 minutes per side, or place on a sheet pan and bake for 25 minutes at 350°. Flip after 15 minutes.

Serves 4

To Balance the Meal: serve 2 sausages and a poached egg on a slice of rye toast with 2 tsp. butter.

To make gluten free:
Cook the egg with 1 c. vegetables in 2 tsp. butter and ½ c. rice in place of rye toast

To make dairy free:
Substitute coconut oil for butter

Zucchini Pancakes

4 eggs - whisked
3 Tbsp. coconut, almond, or cassava flour
1 tsp. dried, or 1 Tbsp. fresh dill
¼ tsp. salt
Pinch of pepper
3 c. shredded zucchini - loosely packed and squeezed of extra liquid
1 Tbsp. coconut or avocado oil for frying

Combine whisked egg with the flour, dill, salt and pepper. Stir in the zucchini.

Heat a large skillet over medium heat and add coconut/avocado oil. Spoon ¼ cup of the batter into the skillet and spread to pancake shape. When bubbles form around the edges, flip and cook until golden brown about 3 minutes per side.

1 Tbsp. sour cream
1 Tbsp. fresh chives - minced

Serve with 1 Tbsp. of sour cream and chives mixed.

Serves 2

To Balance the Meal: serve with 1 oz. Turkey Breakfast Sausages (p. 42) and ½ c. sliced strawberries.

To make gluten free:
This meal is gluten free

To make dairy free:
Substitute a nut butter for the sour cream

The Weight & Wellness Way to a Healthy Weight

Won't I gain weight if I eat this much?

Most people are able to lose those unwanted pounds following the Weight & Wellness Way of eating. People lose body fat, gain muscle mass and improve their metabolism, energy and sense of well-being. They happily report that they are not hungry and have fewer cravings.

In the past, you may have tried to lose weight by reducing fat or calories. However, after those diets, you may have regained the weight you lost or discovered that your metabolism was even slower. At Nutritional Weight & Wellness, we have a better approach. We put the science of weight loss to work for you. Here's how:

- Eating sufficient protein can increase your metabolism by up to 30 percent for several hours.
- Healthy fats provide satiety (a feeling of satisfaction that keeps you full), help stabilize blood sugar and reduce cravings.
- Vegetables, fruits and whole grains, naturally high in fiber, leave you energized far longer than the breads and snacks that quickly break down into sugar in your bloodstream.
- Eating smaller amounts of protein, carbohydrates and healthy fats five to six times per day balances your blood sugar, curbs cravings and gives your body the fuel it needs to burn rather than store calories.

Mary Lou's success story–70 pounds gone, no more prescriptions and feeling great at age 73

Four years ago I was a totally different person. I was overweight, struggled with chronic pain from fibromyalgia and was taking 12 prescription medications for high blood pressure, high cholesterol, GERD, anxiety, sleep problems and pain. The prescriptions left me feeling lethargic and in a fog most of the time. I had trouble moving and relied on my cane to walk.

My daughters encouraged me to have a nutrition counseling appointment with Darlene because I had been experiencing severe stomach issues. I had a lot of pain from IBS and was throwing up. Darlene recommended that I eliminate gluten from my diet. At first, I simply replaced my usual foods with gluten free versions. Over time, I learned that gluten free processed foods still contain unhealthy ingredients, even though they are gluten free. Eventually, I eliminated these products from my diet too.

Then, about a year ago, I enrolled in the ***Nutrition 4 Weight Loss Program*** *with my daughter.* ***The classes taught me great tips such as batch cooking—on the grill and using a crockpot—*** *and how a glass of wine each night isn't as innocent as it seems. I'm so thankful to Darlene and my Nutrition 4 Weight Loss teacher, Angela, for all the things they taught me.* ***I learned how to portion out healthy proteins, carbs and fats in my refrigerator and then assemble meals throughout the week so it's easy for me to stay on track.*** *I still meet with Darlene occasionally for continued support as I get healthier.*

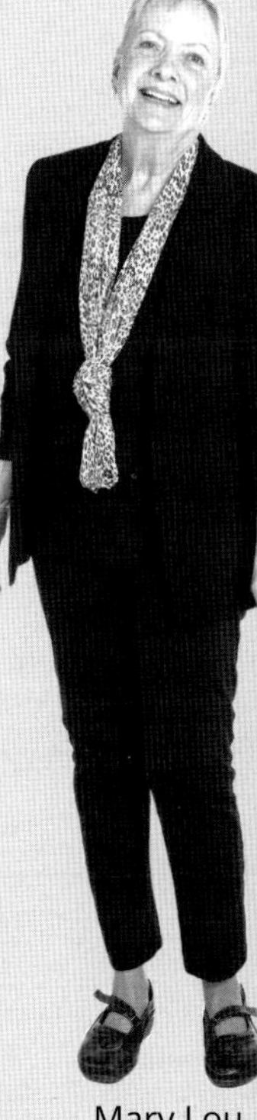

Mary Lou AFTER

I've now lost 70 pounds *and I no longer need a cane to move around. It has been a treat to go into the regular women's department to shop for clothes rather than the plus size section. Best of all,* ***I'm off all the prescription medications I was taking. My blood pressure and cholesterol are normal, my arthritis has improved, I have better digestion, and I'm focused and energized.*** *Five days per week I work out at the gym doing weight-lifting routines, chair yoga classes and more. My doctor has been thrilled with my test results!*

As I reminisce about my husband who passed away three years ago from cancer, I am even more motivated to take care of myself. ***This healthy lifestyle is a gift I've given to myself—to live a longer, happy, active life.***

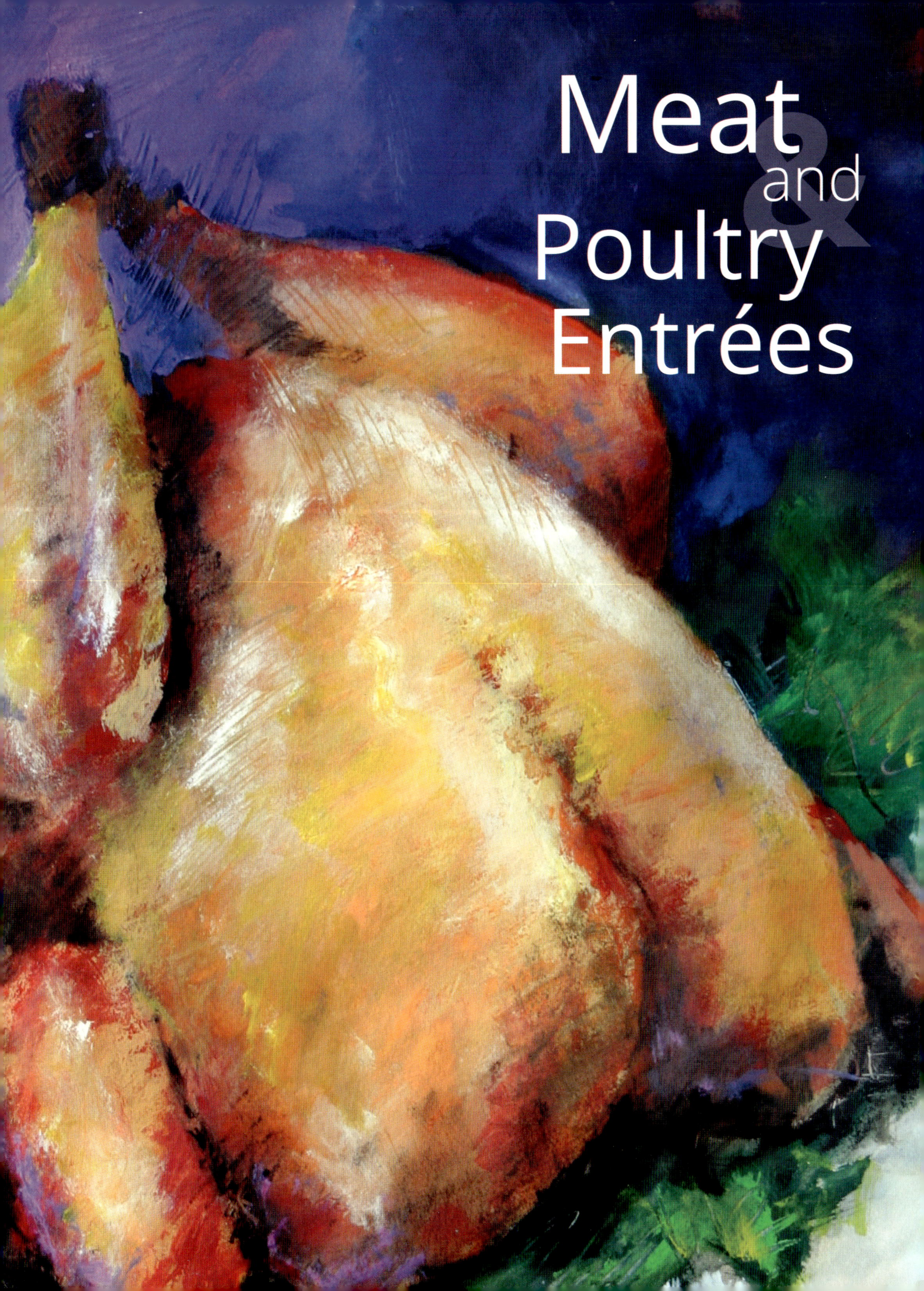

Meat & Poultry Entrées

Beef

Chicken

Pork and Lamb

Turkey

Asian Beef and Vegetables Meal-in-a-Bag

2 cloves garlic - minced
2 lb. ground beef
2 tsp. ginger - grated
1½ tsp. salt
½ tsp. pepper
¼ c. green onion - chopped

Preheat oven to 350º.

Mix together and divide into 6 patties. Place each patty in individual parchment bag*.

2 c. carrots - sliced
6 c. green beans - cut in half
3 c. red bell pepper - sliced
3 c. baby bok choy - chopped
3 Tbsp. avocado oil
2 Tbsp. Bragg Liquid Aminos or coconut aminos
1 tsp. salt

Combine vegetables and toss in olive oil, Bragg Liquid Aminos and salt. Divide evenly into the 6 parchment bags. Place parchment bags on a baking sheet.

Bake at 350º for 40-45 minutes.

Serves 6

To Balance the Meal: this meal is balanced.

To make gluten free:
This is gluten free

To make dairy free:
This is dairy free

** Can use a parchment sheet folded over and creased to seal.*

Beef and Wild Rice Meatloaf

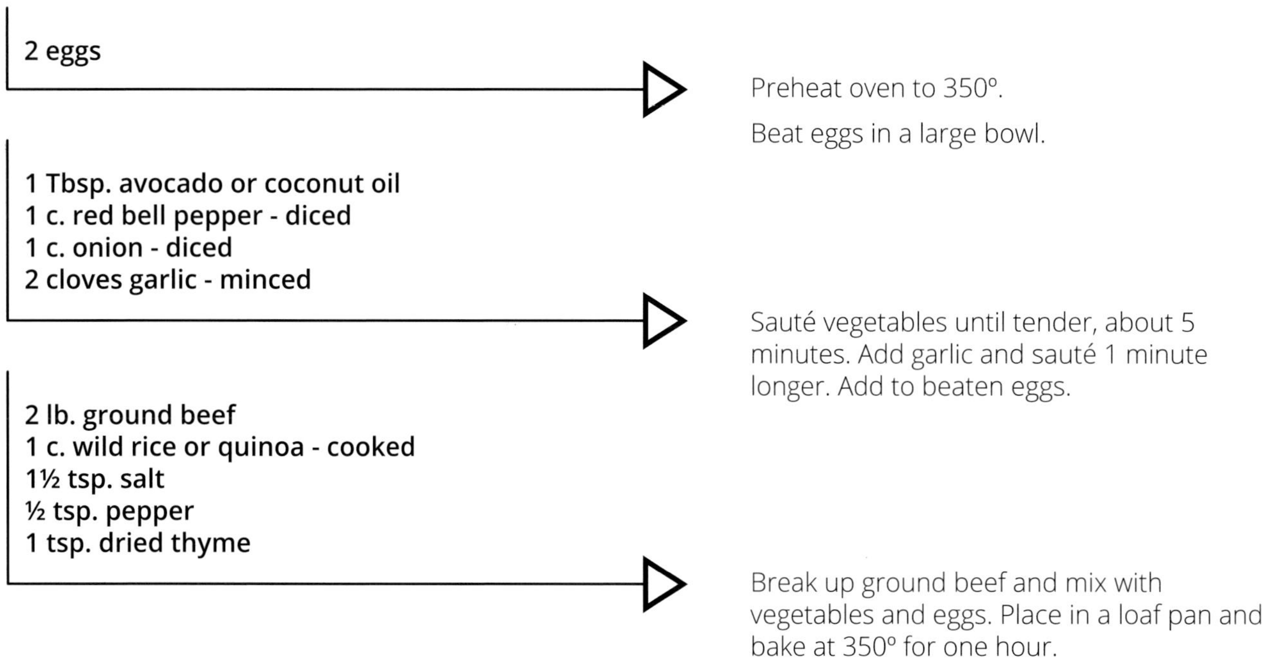

Serves 6

To Balance the Meal: serve with 2 c. green beans or Brussels sprouts and ¼ c. winter squash.

To make gluten free:
This is gluten free

To make dairy free:
This is dairy free

Beef Stir-Fry

2 Tbsp. coconut or avocado oil
2 c. broccoli - cut into bite-sized pieces
1 c. yellow onion - chopped
1 c. carrots - sliced thin
1 red bell pepper - sliced
2 c. pea pods - trimmed or frozen peas
2 garlic cloves - minced
2 tsp. grated ginger (optional)

Heat a large skillet or wok to med-high, add oil and sauté first four vegetables about five minutes (long enough to be slightly cooked but still crunchy). Add the pea pods, garlic and ginger. Cook for 2 minutes more and set aside in a bowl.

1 ½ lbs. sirloin - cut thin, against the grain
¼ tsp. sea salt and pepper to taste

Season beef lightly with salt and pepper. In the same pan, heat oil and briefly sear the beef, being careful not to overcook. Add vegetables back to the pan.

Sauce:
¼ c. Bragg Liquid Aminos or coconut aminos
1 Tbsp. sherry or rice vinegar
2 tsp. toasted sesame oil
Dash cayenne pepper

Combine sauce ingredients in a small bowl and pour over the beef and vegetables. Stir to coat.

2 c. brown basmati rice - cooked
¼ c. green onions - thinly sliced

Add rice and mix thoroughly with the meat and vegetables. Divide into 4 bowls and top with green onions.

Serves 4

To Balance the Meal: this meal is balanced.

To make gluten free:
This meal is gluten free

To make dairy free:
This meal is dairy free

Bison Burger

1½ lb. ground bison meat
½ c. diced onion
1 clove garlic - minced
2 tsp. salt
1 Tbsp. avocado oil

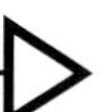

In a large bowl, combine ground bison, onion, garlic, and salt. Mix by hand or with a wooden spoon and form into 4 patties, coat with oil.

Preheat grill. Grill burgers until done.

Serves 4

To Balance the Meal: serve with 1-2 c. green beans and Sweet Potato Wedges (p. 155).

To make gluten free:
This is gluten free

To make dairy free:
This is dairy free

Bison or Beef Shepherd's Pie

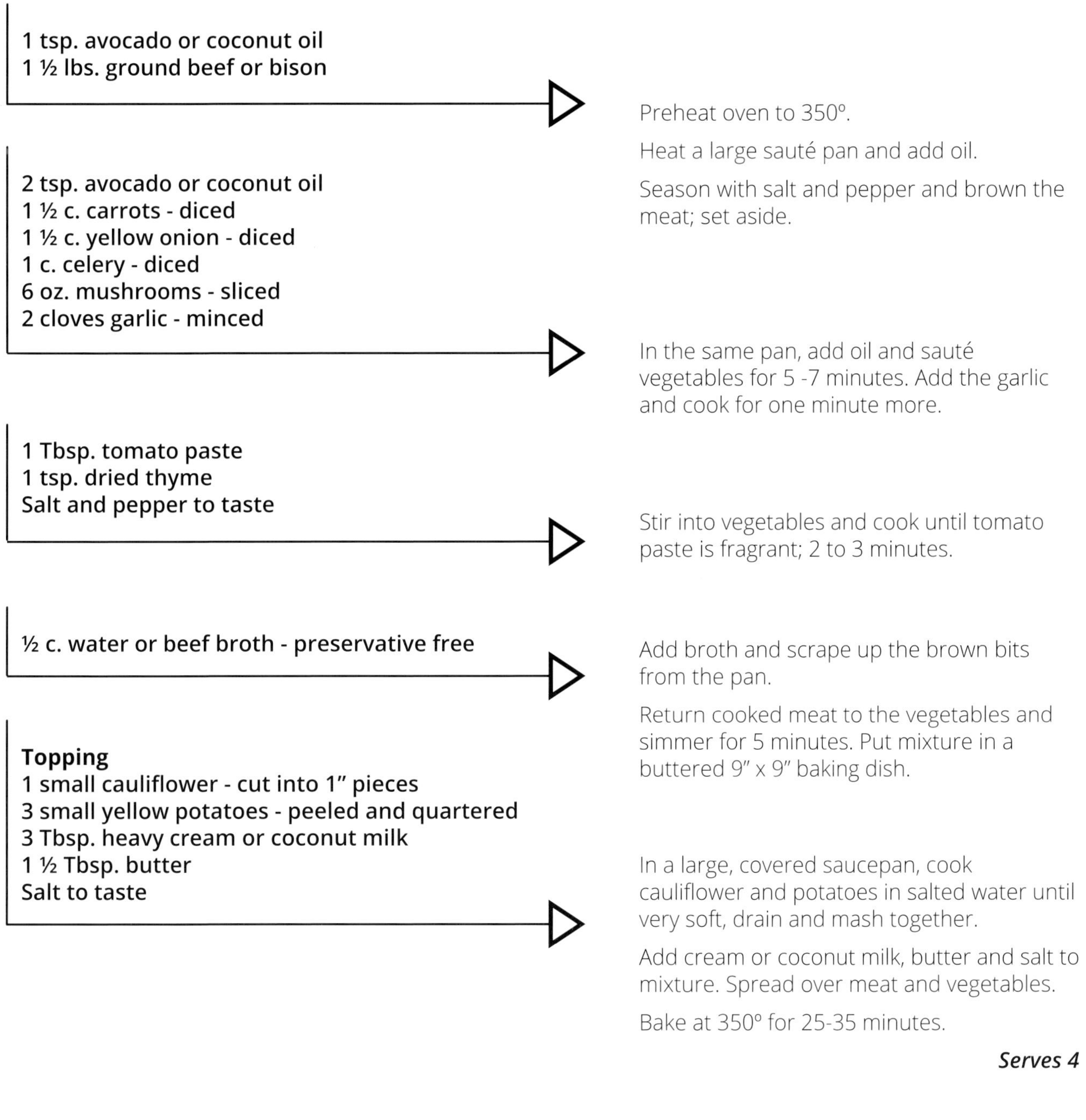

1 tsp. avocado or coconut oil
1 ½ lbs. ground beef or bison

Preheat oven to 350º.

Heat a large sauté pan and add oil.

Season with salt and pepper and brown the meat; set aside.

2 tsp. avocado or coconut oil
1 ½ c. carrots - diced
1 ½ c. yellow onion - diced
1 c. celery - diced
6 oz. mushrooms - sliced
2 cloves garlic - minced

In the same pan, add oil and sauté vegetables for 5 -7 minutes. Add the garlic and cook for one minute more.

1 Tbsp. tomato paste
1 tsp. dried thyme
Salt and pepper to taste

Stir into vegetables and cook until tomato paste is fragrant; 2 to 3 minutes.

½ c. water or beef broth - preservative free

Add broth and scrape up the brown bits from the pan.

Return cooked meat to the vegetables and simmer for 5 minutes. Put mixture in a buttered 9" x 9" baking dish.

Topping
1 small cauliflower - cut into 1" pieces
3 small yellow potatoes - peeled and quartered
3 Tbsp. heavy cream or coconut milk
1 ½ Tbsp. butter
Salt to taste

In a large, covered saucepan, cook cauliflower and potatoes in salted water until very soft, drain and mash together.

Add cream or coconut milk, butter and salt to mixture. Spread over meat and vegetables.

Bake at 350º for 25-35 minutes.

Serves 4

To Balance the Meal: this is a balanced meal.

To make gluten free:
This is gluten free

To make dairy free:
Use coconut milk and olive oil in place of cream and butter

Chili

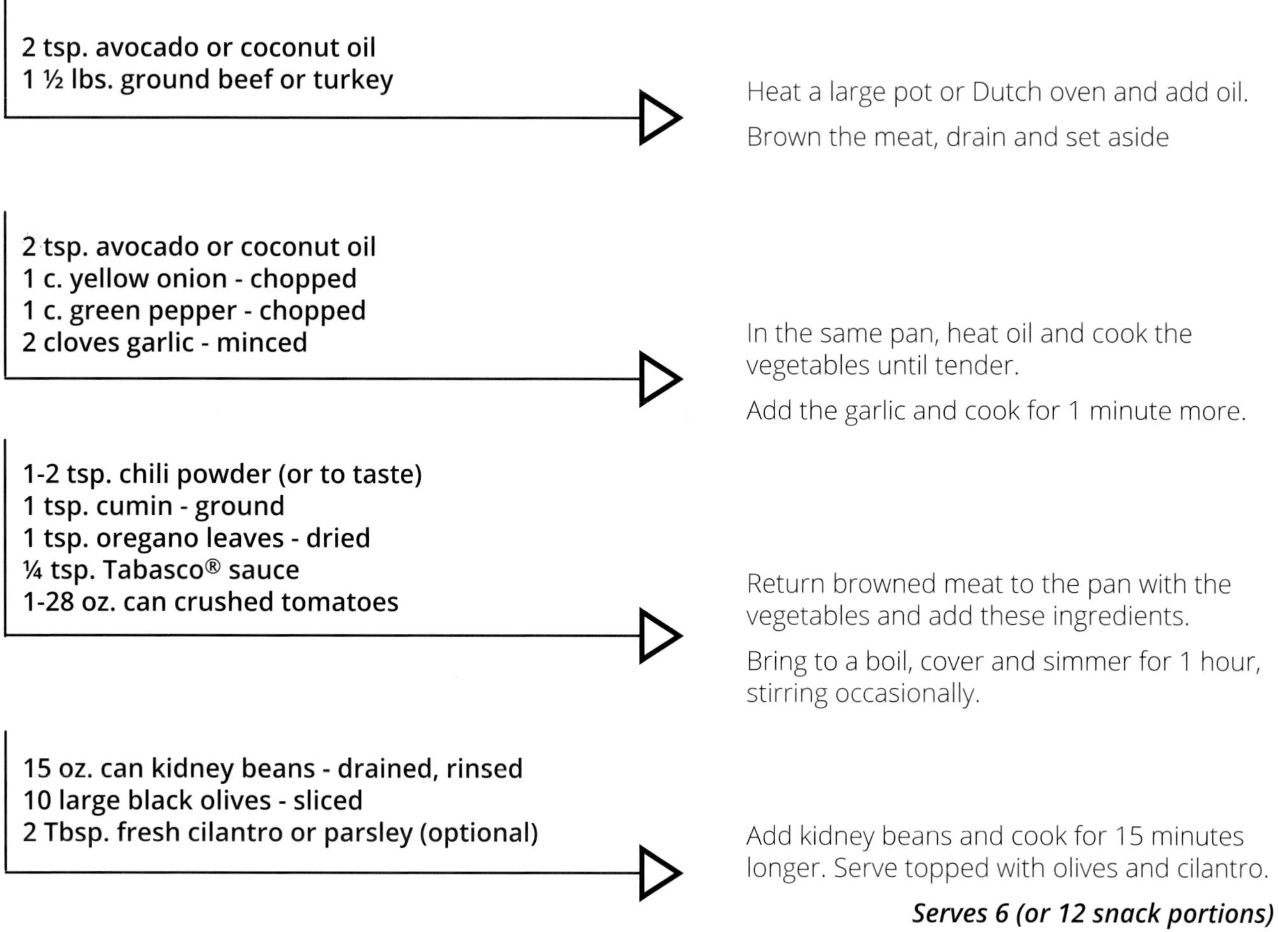

2 tsp. avocado or coconut oil
1 ½ lbs. ground beef or turkey

Heat a large pot or Dutch oven and add oil.

Brown the meat, drain and set aside

2 tsp. avocado or coconut oil
1 c. yellow onion - chopped
1 c. green pepper - chopped
2 cloves garlic - minced

In the same pan, heat oil and cook the vegetables until tender.

Add the garlic and cook for 1 minute more.

1-2 tsp. chili powder (or to taste)
1 tsp. cumin - ground
1 tsp. oregano leaves - dried
¼ tsp. Tabasco® sauce
1-28 oz. can crushed tomatoes

Return browned meat to the pan with the vegetables and add these ingredients.

Bring to a boil, cover and simmer for 1 hour, stirring occasionally.

15 oz. can kidney beans - drained, rinsed
10 large black olives - sliced
2 Tbsp. fresh cilantro or parsley (optional)

Add kidney beans and cook for 15 minutes longer. Serve topped with olives and cilantro.

Serves 6 (or 12 snack portions)

To Balance the Meal: serve 2 c. chili with 2 c. romaine leaves, 1 c. fresh salad vegetables and 1 Tbsp. olive oil dressing or ½ c. rice and 1 Tbsp. sour cream.

To make gluten free:
This is gluten free

To make dairy free:
This is dairy free

Crockpot® Chuck Roast

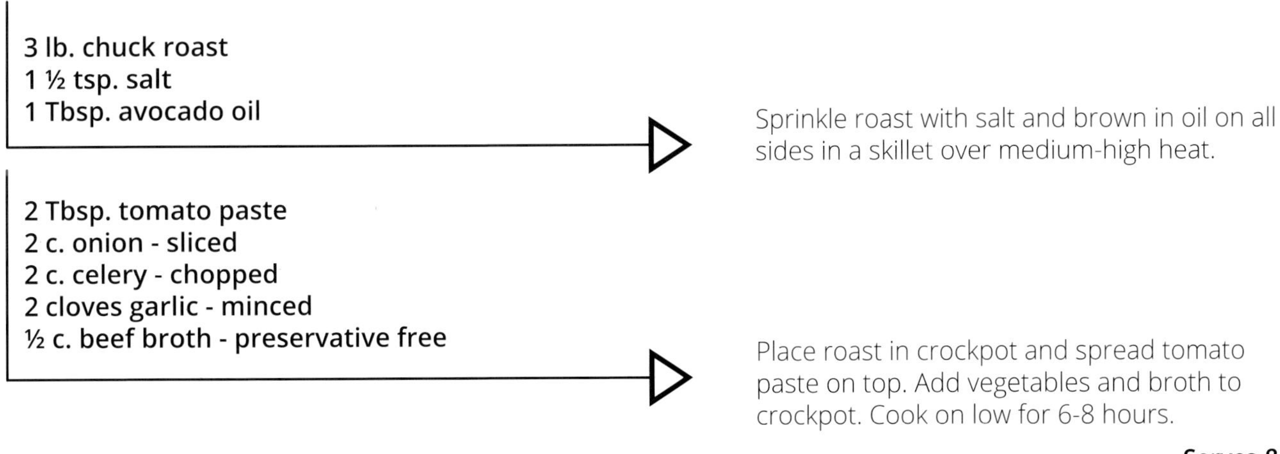

3 lb. chuck roast
1 ½ tsp. salt
1 Tbsp. avocado oil

Sprinkle roast with salt and brown in oil on all sides in a skillet over medium-high heat.

2 Tbsp. tomato paste
2 c. onion - sliced
2 c. celery - chopped
2 cloves garlic - minced
½ c. beef broth - preservative free

Place roast in crockpot and spread tomato paste on top. Add vegetables and broth to crockpot. Cook on low for 6-8 hours.

Serves 8

To Balance the Meal: serve 4 oz. roast with ½ c. boiled potato or ½ c. steamed carrots with 2 tsp. butter.

To make gluten free:
This is gluten free

To make dairy free:
Substitute coconut oil for butter

Deep Dish Pizza Pie

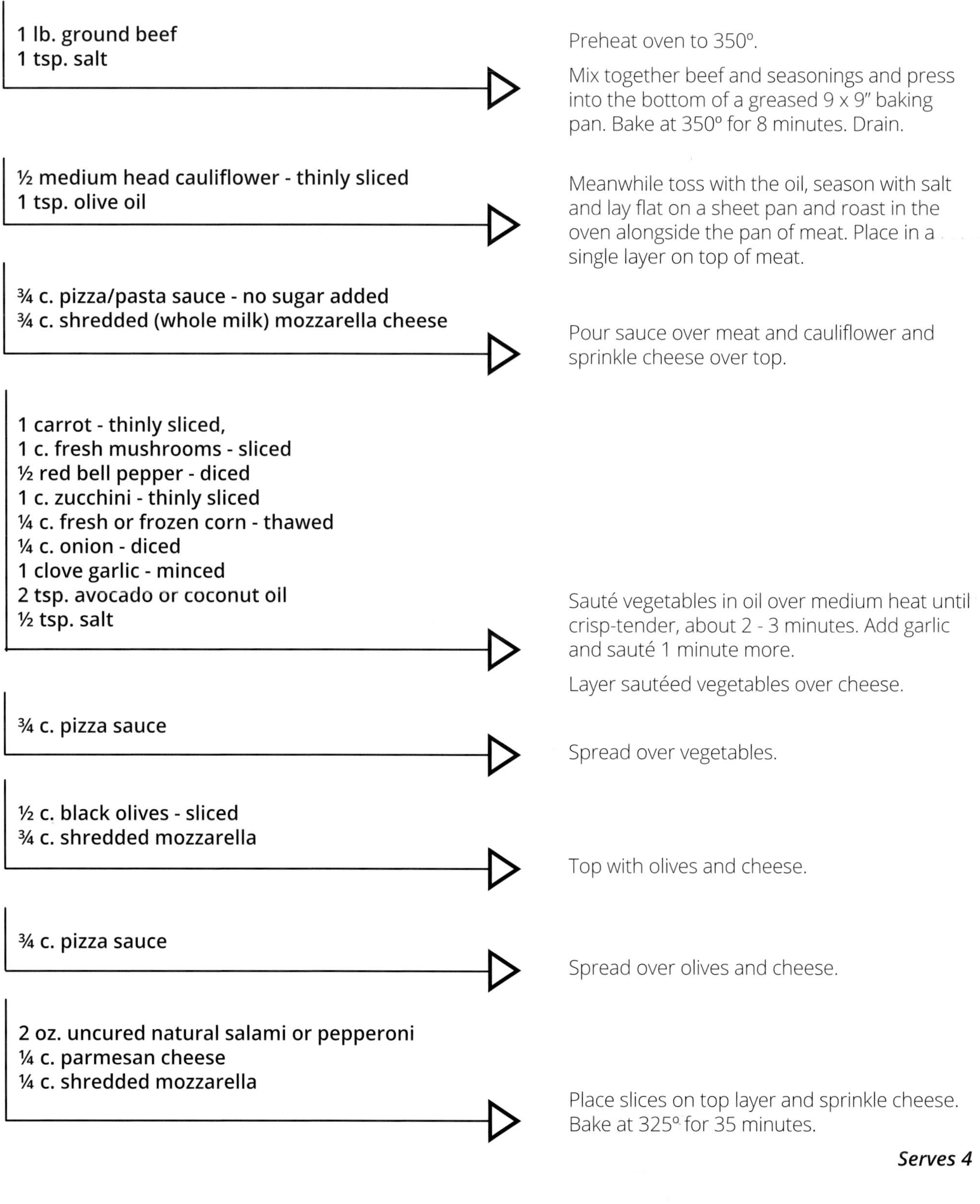

1 lb. ground beef
1 tsp. salt

Preheat oven to 350º.

Mix together beef and seasonings and press into the bottom of a greased 9 x 9" baking pan. Bake at 350º for 8 minutes. Drain.

½ medium head cauliflower - thinly sliced
1 tsp. olive oil

Meanwhile toss with the oil, season with salt and lay flat on a sheet pan and roast in the oven alongside the pan of meat. Place in a single layer on top of meat.

¾ c. pizza/pasta sauce - no sugar added
¾ c. shredded (whole milk) mozzarella cheese

Pour sauce over meat and cauliflower and sprinkle cheese over top.

1 carrot - thinly sliced,
1 c. fresh mushrooms - sliced
½ red bell pepper - diced
1 c. zucchini - thinly sliced
¼ c. fresh or frozen corn - thawed
¼ c. onion - diced
1 clove garlic - minced
2 tsp. avocado or coconut oil
½ tsp. salt

Sauté vegetables in oil over medium heat until crisp-tender, about 2 - 3 minutes. Add garlic and sauté 1 minute more.

Layer sautéed vegetables over cheese.

¾ c. pizza sauce

Spread over vegetables.

½ c. black olives - sliced
¾ c. shredded mozzarella

Top with olives and cheese.

¾ c. pizza sauce

Spread over olives and cheese.

2 oz. uncured natural salami or pepperoni
¼ c. parmesan cheese
¼ c. shredded mozzarella

Place slices on top layer and sprinkle cheese. Bake at 325º for 35 minutes.

Serves 4

To make gluten free:
This is gluten free

To make dairy free:
Cannot be made dairy free

Grilled Grass-Fed Steak

4, 5-8 oz. grass-fed steaks (T-bone, skirt, ribeye, flank, strip, sirloin)
2 Tbsp. melted organic butter
Salt and pepper to taste

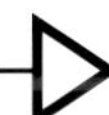

Preheat grill to medium heat and brush each steak with melted butter and dust with salt and black pepper.

Depending upon thickness of steak, grill each side for 4-6 minutes. To ensure steaks stay moist, do not overcook. Cooking beyond medium done will dry out the steaks.

Allow the steaks to rest 10 minutes before serving.

Serves 4

To Balance the Meal: serve with 2 c. of grilled vegetables tossed in olive oil.

To make gluten free:
This is gluten free

To make dairy free:
Substitute coconut oil for butter

Fact *VS.* **Fiction**

Fiction	Fact
It doesn't matter if meat is organic. They just say it is organic so they can charge more.	Animals that have been raised organically cannot be given hormones or unnecessary antibiotics. Today, 70 percent of all antibiotics are used for animals, which contributes to problems of antibiotic resistance in people. Meat from animals that are commercially raised in confined settings contain hormone and antibiotic residue that can lead to weight gain in people, just like it does for animals.

Sloppy Joes

1½ tsp. salt
1 Tbsp. avocado oil
½ c. onion - diced
1 c. celery - diced
1 c. red pepper - diced
½ c. carrots - diced
2 cloves garlic - diced

Sauté vegetables in oil until tender. Season with salt.

1½ lb. ground beef or turkey

Add beef or turkey to vegetables, use a fork to crumble the meat.

1 c. tomato sauce - preservative and sugar free
¼ c. organic ketchup
1 Tbsp. yellow mustard
½ tsp. black pepper

Add to meat and vegetables and cook through.

Serves 4

To Balance the Meal: serve on a whole grain bun with 2 c. steamed vegetables.

To make gluten free:
Use a gluten-free bun or vegetable option

To make dairy free:
This is dairy free

Fact *VS.* **Fiction**

Fiction	Fact
If chips say "no refined oils," they are OK to eat.	Even if a food claims to have no damaged fats, check the food label for the words hydrogenated or partially hydrogenated oils. Often the serving size is 4 chips or less to stay within the limit to claim the food has no damaged fats.

Wild Rice Meatballs

1¼ lb. ground beef
1 egg - slightly beaten
½ c. onion - finely chopped
1 c. wild rice - cooked
1 tsp. salt
1 tsp. garlic powder or finely chopped garlic

Preheat oven to 375º.

Combine ingredients and shape into 12 meatballs, approximately 1½" in diameter.

Place on baking sheet.

Bake 30-40 minutes or until brown.

Serves 4

To Balance the Meal: serve with 2 c. green beans, ½ c. sweet potatoes with 2 tsp. butter.

To make gluten free:
This meal is gluten free

To make dairy free:
Use coconut oil instead of butter

The Weight & Wellness Way to Reduce Pain and Inflammation

Madeline's success story—30 years of back pain gone and a new zest for life gained

When I think about the 30 years I struggled with back pain, it brings me to tears. I missed out on so much including my daughter's college graduation when I ended up in the hospital and my father's eightieth birthday celebration when I couldn't do anything other than stand up straight and still because I was in so much pain. ***My back pain ruled my life. When I had back spasms, I couldn't sit, lie down or move; many times I couldn't work. I could only stand still and ride out the pain.*** *I sought out help from chiropractors, acupuncturists, massage therapists, and physical therapists, which provided only temporary relief.*

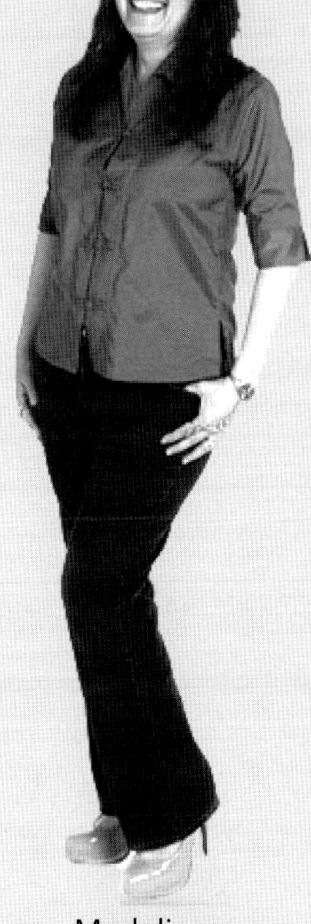
Madeline

My pain got to be so debilitating that my doctor recommended that I have a device implanted in my spine that would "trick" my body into not feeling the pain. This made no sense to me because I knew it wouldn't solve the cause of my pain. If I could resolve the cause, there wouldn't be any pain. But I had to do something since I was already taking four pain pills per day, and my doctor said that over time I would need even more pain medication to keep the pain away. And because of the back pain, I was only getting two to three hours of sleep each night. The lack of sleep left me feeling anxious and irritable, and my memory was awful. The pain pills caused chronic constipation and heartburn, and my hair was falling out in clumps. Before moving forward with the drastic surgery, I decided to try one more thing...nutrition. I figured I didn't have anything to lose.

I had been a long-time listener of the **Dishing Up Nutrition** *radio show and decided to make a nutrition counseling appointment. At my first appointment with Darlene, I told her my goals were to be drug free and pain free; and within two months, Darlene delivered. Darlene designed a careful eating plan for me that addressed certain food sensitivities that were contributing to my pain.* ***Until I came to Nutritional Weight & Wellness, no one had been able to find the source of my back pain, and I had dealt with doctors and all sorts of therapies for over 30 years.***

I do occasionally miss some of the foods I used to eat such as pizza, bagels, milk and ice cream. But when I think of how much pain I was in and of how far I've come, it's easy for me to pass on eating these foods. My heart breaks when I think back on all the things I missed because of my back pain. I was depressed because of all the pain that I was feeling and never want to feel that bad again; no food would ever be worth it.

I am now off all of my pain medications and haven't had a back spasm in over a year (since I started seeing Darlene). I am able to bounce out of bed in the morning after seven hours of pain-free sleep! My anxiety and constipation are gone and my memory is much better. *On top of everything, I lost 30 pounds! I wasn't aiming to lose any weight, but it's been a nice side effect of the new eating plan.* ***I feel like a new, younger person. It feels wonderful to not hurt anymore!***

Cheesy Broccoli and Chicken Casserole

1¼ lb. chicken breast - boneless and skinless
12 oz. bag pre-cut broccoli

Preheat oven to 400º.

Bring a large pot of water to a boil and add the chicken breasts. Simmer 15 minutes.

Add broccoli to water and continue to simmer 3 minutes. Drain and set aside. Cool chicken and cut into bite-size pieces.

4 strips of bacon

Brown the bacon in a skillet then place on paper towels to drain.

5 eggs
½ c. heavy cream
1 c. whole milk
¼ c. almond flour or corn meal
2 tsp. black pepper
½ tsp. salt
1 Tbsp. Dijon mustard
½ c. grated cheddar or mozzarella cheese

Butter a 9x9" casserole dish.

In a large bowl, whisk together the eggs, cream, milk, almond flour, pepper, salt, and mustard. Stir in cheese.

Place the broccoli and chicken in the greased casserole dish.

Pour egg mixture over the broccoli and chicken.

½ c. grated cheddar or mozzarella cheese

Crumble bacon over the top and then sprinkle with the remaining cheese.

Bake at 400º for 30-45 minutes until set and top is browned.

Serves 5

To Balance the Meal: serve with a large side salad and 1 tsp. olive oil.

To make gluten free:
This is gluten free

To make dairy free:
This cannot be made dairy free

Chicken and Brussels Sprouts in Sun-Dried Tomatoes

8 oz. sun-dried tomatoes in olive oil - sliced
1½ tsp. salt
2 tsp. dried basil
½ c. chicken broth - preservative free

Preheat oven to 350°.

Mix together in a small bowl.

2 lb. boneless skinless chicken thighs or breasts
2 c. Brussels sprouts - halved
2 c. cauliflower - cut into bite-size pieces
2 c. broccoli - cut into bite-size pieces

Combine chicken and vegetables in a 13" x 9" baking dish. Pour tomato/oil mixture over chicken and vegetables.

Toss to coat. Bake at 350° for 45-50 minutes.

Serves 6

To Balance the Meal: serve with ½ c. brown rice.

To make gluten free:
This is gluten free

To make dairy free:
This is dairy free

Chicken and Potato Enchiladas

2 c. red potatoes - thinly sliced
½ tsp. salt

Preheat oven to 350° degrees.

In a saucepan, bring water, salt and potatoes to a boil. Reduce heat and simmer until just tender, about 3-4 minutes

2 Tbsp. avocado oil
½ tsp. salt
2 lb. chicken breast or thighs - cut into bite-size pieces

Season the chicken with salt and heat oil in a large sauté pan. Brown the chicken for 4 - 5 minutes.

Sauce
1 c. salsa
1 c. tomato sauce
1 Tbsp. chili powder
2 tsp. cumin
2 tsp. dried oregano
1 c. chicken broth - preservative free
½ tsp. salt

Combine sauce ingredients with the chicken. Simmer for about 10 minutes, stirring occasionally.

1 c. shredded cheese

In an oiled, square baking dish layer: sauce/chicken, potatoes, sauce/chicken, potatoes, sauce/chicken. Top with shredded cheese. Bake at 350° for 30-40 minutes until hot and bubbly.

Serves 6

To Balance the Meal: this is a balanced meal.

To make gluten free:
This is gluten free

To make dairy free:
This cannot be made dairy free

Chicken with Spaghetti Squash & Pasta

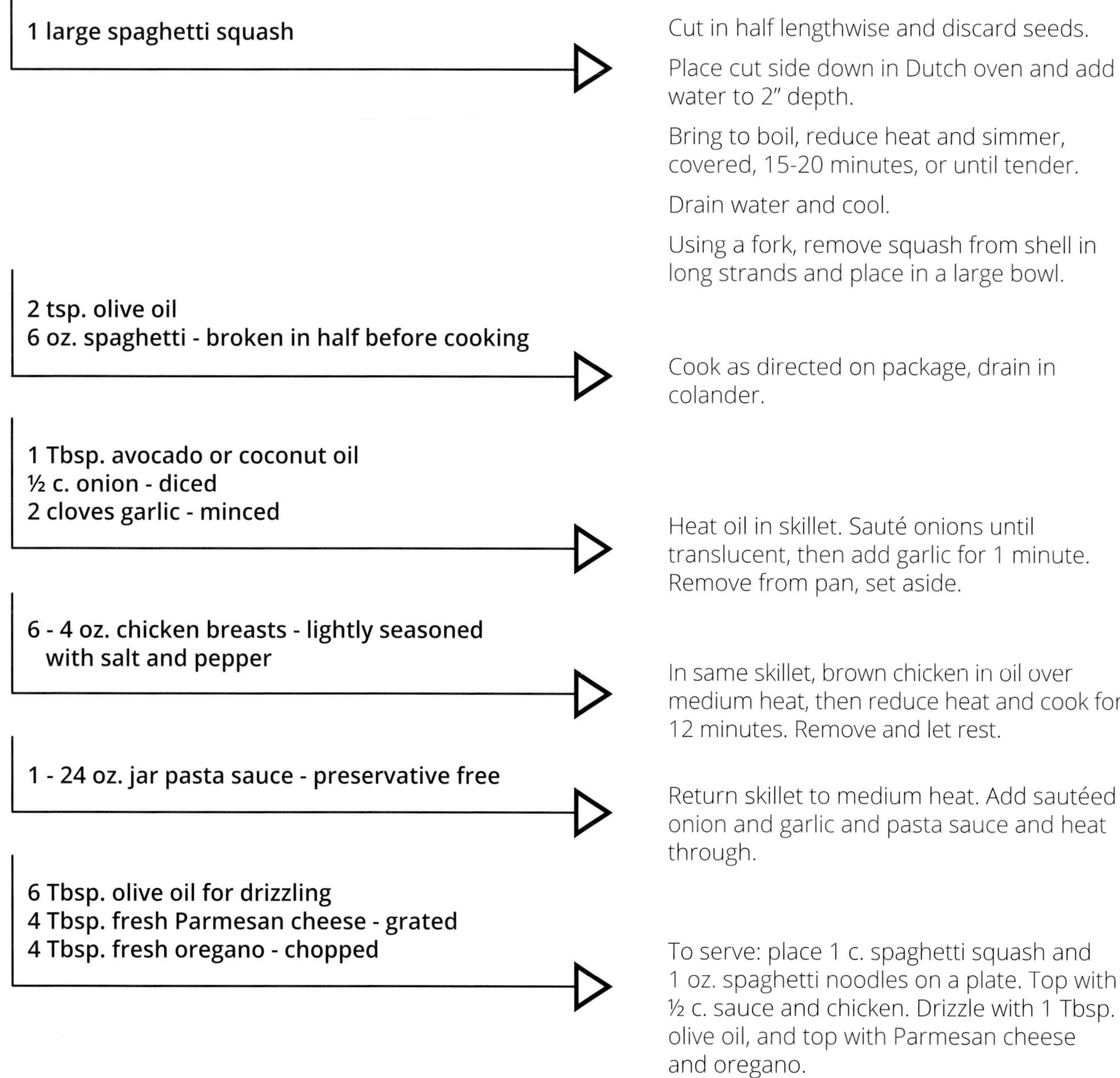

1 large spaghetti squash

Cut in half lengthwise and discard seeds.

Place cut side down in Dutch oven and add water to 2" depth.

Bring to boil, reduce heat and simmer, covered, 15-20 minutes, or until tender.

Drain water and cool.

Using a fork, remove squash from shell in long strands and place in a large bowl.

2 tsp. olive oil
6 oz. spaghetti - broken in half before cooking

Cook as directed on package, drain in colander.

1 Tbsp. avocado or coconut oil
½ c. onion - diced
2 cloves garlic - minced

Heat oil in skillet. Sauté onions until translucent, then add garlic for 1 minute. Remove from pan, set aside.

6 - 4 oz. chicken breasts - lightly seasoned with salt and pepper

In same skillet, brown chicken in oil over medium heat, then reduce heat and cook for 12 minutes. Remove and let rest.

1 - 24 oz. jar pasta sauce - preservative free

Return skillet to medium heat. Add sautéed onion and garlic and pasta sauce and heat through.

6 Tbsp. olive oil for drizzling
4 Tbsp. fresh Parmesan cheese - grated
4 Tbsp. fresh oregano - chopped

To serve: place 1 c. spaghetti squash and 1 oz. spaghetti noodles on a plate. Top with ½ c. sauce and chicken. Drizzle with 1 Tbsp. olive oil, and top with Parmesan cheese and oregano.

Serves 6

To Balance the Meal: serve with 4 c. mixed greens tossed with 1-2 Tbsp. Simple Salad Dressing (p.134).

To make gluten free:
Use gluten-free spaghetti

To make dairy free:
Omit the cheese

Chicken Stir-Fry

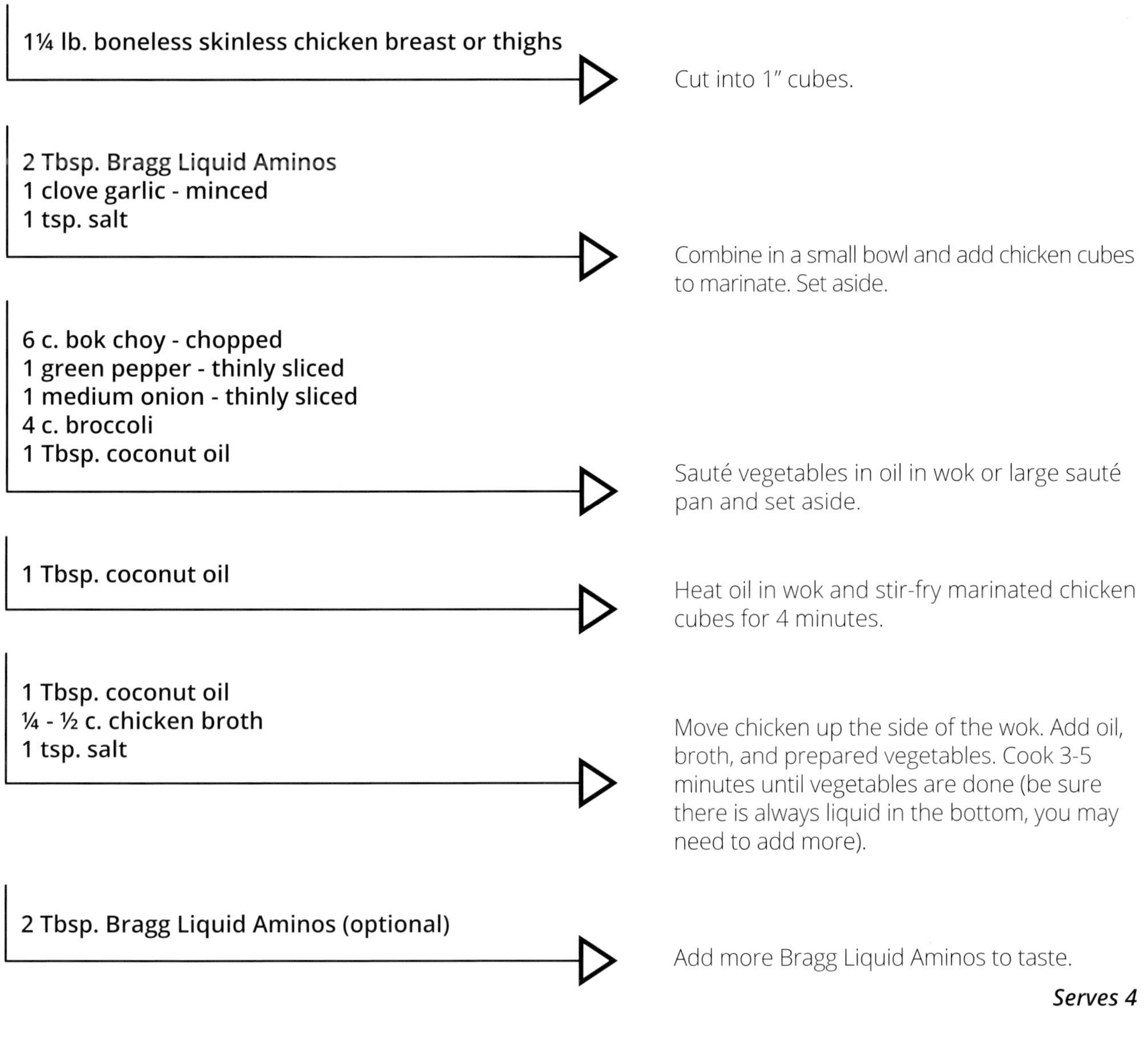

1¼ lb. boneless skinless chicken breast or thighs

Cut into 1" cubes.

2 Tbsp. Bragg Liquid Aminos
1 clove garlic - minced
1 tsp. salt

Combine in a small bowl and add chicken cubes to marinate. Set aside.

6 c. bok choy - chopped
1 green pepper - thinly sliced
1 medium onion - thinly sliced
4 c. broccoli
1 Tbsp. coconut oil

Sauté vegetables in oil in wok or large sauté pan and set aside.

1 Tbsp. coconut oil

Heat oil in wok and stir-fry marinated chicken cubes for 4 minutes.

1 Tbsp. coconut oil
¼ - ½ c. chicken broth
1 tsp. salt

Move chicken up the side of the wok. Add oil, broth, and prepared vegetables. Cook 3-5 minutes until vegetables are done (be sure there is always liquid in the bottom, you may need to add more).

2 Tbsp. Bragg Liquid Aminos (optional)

Add more Bragg Liquid Aminos to taste.

Serves 4

To Balance the Meal: serve over ½ c. brown rice with 2 Tbsp. slivered almonds on top.

To make gluten free:
This meal is gluten free

To make dairy free:
This meal is dairy free

Chicken and Vegetables Meal-in-a-Bag

1 Tbsp olive oil
¼ c. parsley
1 clove garlic - minced
¼ c. onion - diced
1½ tsp. salt
½ tsp. pepper
2 lb. chicken breast or thighs - boneless, skinless

Preheat oven to 350º.

Mix together and divide into 6 portions. Place in individual parchment bags*.

2 red peppers - cut into thick strips
6 c. broccoli - cut into bite-size pieces
3 c. carrots or parsnips - sliced
6 c. cauliflower - cut into bite-size pieces
3 Tbsp. olive oil
1½ tsp. salt
1 Tbsp. fresh thyme or rosemary - chopped

Combine vegetables and mix in olive oil and salt. Divide vegetables evenly into the 6 parchment bags and place parchment bags on a baking sheet.

Bake at 350° for 40-45 minutes.

Serves 6

To Balance the Meal: this meal is balanced

To make gluten free:
This is gluten free

To make dairy free:
This is dairy free

** Can use a parchment sheet folded over and creased to seal.*

Chicken Zucchini Bake

2 Tbsp. avocado oil
1 clove garlic - minced
1 ¼ lb. boneless, skinless chicken - breast or thighs
1 Tbsp. Italian seasoning
1 ½ tsp. salt - divided
Pepper to taste

Preheat oven to 375º.

In a 13 x 9" baking dish, add the oil and garlic. Place the chicken in the bottom of the dish and season with Italian seasoning, 1 tsp. salt and pepper.

2 c. zucchini - cubed
1 c. cherry tomatoes - halved
1 c. onion - chopped
1 c .celery- chopped
2 c. bell peppers (red or green) - chopped
15 oz. organic tomato sauce

Scatter the vegetables over the chicken and pour the tomato sauce over everything, season with the remaining salt and stir to combine.

1/4 c. fresh parsley or basil - chopped

Bake for 35-40 minutes, until chicken is cooked through. Garnish with fresh herbs.

Serves 4

To Balance the Meal: serve with ½ c. brown rice.

To make gluten free:
This meal is gluten free

To make dairy free:
This meal is dairy free

Crockpot® Chicken Drummies

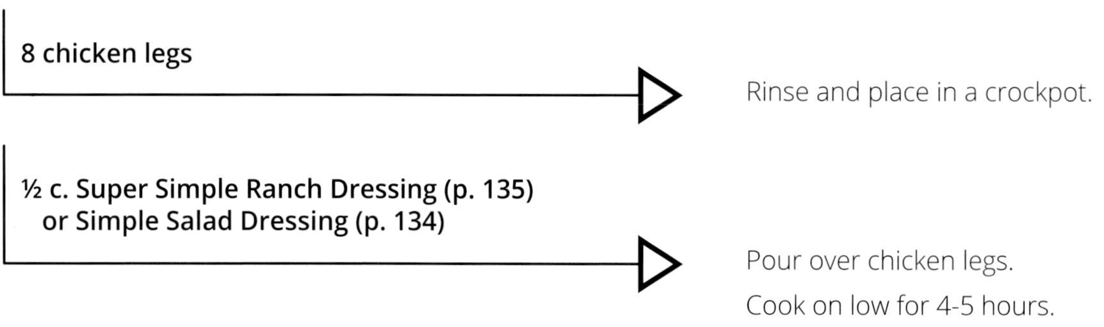

8 chicken legs

Rinse and place in a crockpot.

½ c. Super Simple Ranch Dressing (p. 135) or Simple Salad Dressing (p. 134)

Pour over chicken legs.

Cook on low for 4-5 hours.

Serves 4

To Balance the Meal: serve with 2 c. fresh sliced vegetables and ¼ c. hummus.

To make gluten free:
This is gluten free

To make dairy free:
Use vinaigrette instead of ranch dressing

Fact *VS.* **Fiction**

Fiction	Fact
Eating sugar is normal. What's so bad about drinking soda? It's harmless.	In the 1800s people consumed 2 tsp. of sugar per day. Today we consume 22 tsp. on average. The American Heart Association recommends 6 tsp. or less of sugar per day, for optimal health. Compare that to a can of soda which contains almost 10 tsp. of sugar. That's above and beyond what your body needs for the entire day.

Crockpot® Mexican Chicken Wraps

3 lbs. chicken thighs
1½ c. salsa
1½ tsp. cumin - ground
1½ tsp. salt
1 tsp. oregano - dried

Place chicken in crockpot, top with salsa, and spices. Cook on low for 8 hours.

Shred the cooked chicken with a fork.

Romaine leaves
3 c. corn - fresh or frozen
6 Tbsp. sour cream
1½ avocados
3 Tbsp. red onion - chopped
cilantro - chopped (optional)

For each serving, divide 4 oz. shredded chicken, ½ c. corn, 1 Tbsp. sour cream and ¼ avocado among a few romaine leaves. Eat like a taco. Garnish with onion and cilantro.

Serves 6

To Balance the Meal: this meal is balanced.

To make gluten free:
This is gluten free

To make dairy free:
Omit the sour cream
and add 12 black olives

Be a Deli Detective: What's Hiding in Your Dinner Tonight?

When life gets busy and time is short, it is wonderful to be able to grab a quick and easy pre-made meal from the store, but do you know the ingredients in the foods you choose?

Often times, deli items are not clearly labeled with the ingredients: think hot soups or cold salads at the deli bar. Other times you are in such a rush you may not have time to bother checking the label, so we decided to do the label reading work for you!

	Supermarket	Upscale Grocery Store	Natural Foods Grocery Store	Local Food Co-op
Rotisserie Chicken ingredients:	Sodium phosphate, dextrose, natural flavor, carrageenan	Sodium phosphate, natural flavor	Plain flavor is just chicken! No oil or seasoning, but "Traditional Plain" has canola oil	Plain flavor is salt, pepper and locally-sourced chicken
Mashed Potatoes ingredients:	Butter flavor, dextrose, potassium sorbate, sodium benzoate	Potassium sorbate, mono and diglycerides, sodium diphosphate	Potatoes, butter, milk, salt, pepper	Potatoes, garlic, butter, milk, salt, pepper
Green Beans ingredients:	Not offered at deli	Corn oil, citric acid, phosphoric acid	Beans, garlic, shoyu, expeller-pressed canola oil	Beans, garlic, almonds, lemon juice, expeller-pressed canola oil

We visited several local grocery stores and compared a similar pre-made meal from each location. We were shocked by some of the hidden ingredients in brand names we trusted and thought to be high quality. **The chart above highlights some of the ingredients in each store's products.**

Breaking down the ingredient list

As you can see, **most store-bought deli foods are hiding some ingredients that are unhealthy**. Let's look at each deli item for a thorough understanding of the ingredients.

Rotisserie chicken

Although none of the stores use organic meat for their rotisserie chickens, the natural foods grocery store and the local food co-op use chickens that are free of antibiotics. The co-op is the only one using locally sourced, free range chicken.

The supermarket and upscale grocery stores do not use antibiotic-free meats, and these companies list "natural flavor" on their ingredient labels. **Sometimes "natural flavor" is a hidden term for monosodium glutamate (MSG), which** can cause reactions such as migraines or sleep problems for some people. At the upscale grocery store, the same rotisserie chicken is also packaged and sold already pulled from the bone. This pre-pulled, packaged chicken label includes hydrolyzed soy protein, another possible form of hidden MSG. Interestingly, at the upscale grocery store, all rotisserie chickens are coated with their signature seasoning rub, which also contains natural flavor, leaving us concerned about consuming any of the rotisserie meats there.

The natural foods grocery store offers a pure plain chicken, but be aware that their "Traditional Plain" chicken also contains canola oil. The local food co-op offers a pure plain chicken as well.

Mashed potatoes

Unfortunately, the mashed potatoes are not as pure as expected. Both the supermarket and the upscale grocery store have added preservatives for increased shelf life, color retention, and flavor. The upscale grocery store sells mashed potatoes in both the deli case and pre-packaged to go. The same potatoes are used in each product, yet those in a big bowl behind the glass case contain: potatoes, skim milk, and margarine, while the prepackaged label reads: potatoes, skim milk, butter, as well as all the additives mentioned in the above chart. There is no way to know which label represents the actual mashed potato ingredients, yet neither label represents a very good product.

The natural foods grocery store and local food co-op mashed potatoes says "potatoes only" on the label.

Green beans

Green beans are the vegetable we selected for comparison because we assumed that most stores would carry them. However, the only deli vegetable option that we found at the supermarket was a creamy coleslaw containing high fructose corn syrup and a list of other additives. The green beans at the upscale grocery store are packaged under their new "Modern Plate" label, which is advertised as "nutritionist approved" dishes. The front label reads: "tender green beans braised with fresh garlic and tossed with toasted almonds." Sounds great, right? Upon further investigation—turning the package over to read the ingredients list—we found corn oil and phosphoric acid added to the mix. The upscale grocery store green bean almandine deli label reads: "green beans steamed and mixed with garlic, almonds, salt and pepper," but the ingredients list an olive oil blend, rather than pure olive oil, used in the beans. At the deli, when we asked what kind of canola oil is used in the beans, we were unable to get an answer.

The natural foods grocery store and local food co-op's green beans are made with high quality expeller-pressed canola oil which makes them OK choices.

The bottom line on deli dinners

Overall, the natural foods grocery store and the local food co-op produce items closest to home-cooked real food. In truth, nothing compares to making food in your own home. When you must eat out, the key to choosing high quality, health-promoting prepared foods is to be sure you know the ingredients. If ingredients are not posted in clear view, or you are unsure of what may be hiding inside the product, ask someone. If you cannot get a clear answer, steer clear of that option, and choose another. Being a safe and savvy shopper takes time and energy, which is why we, your Deli Detectives, are on the case helping you discover what may be hiding in your dinner tonight.

Easy Almond Chicken

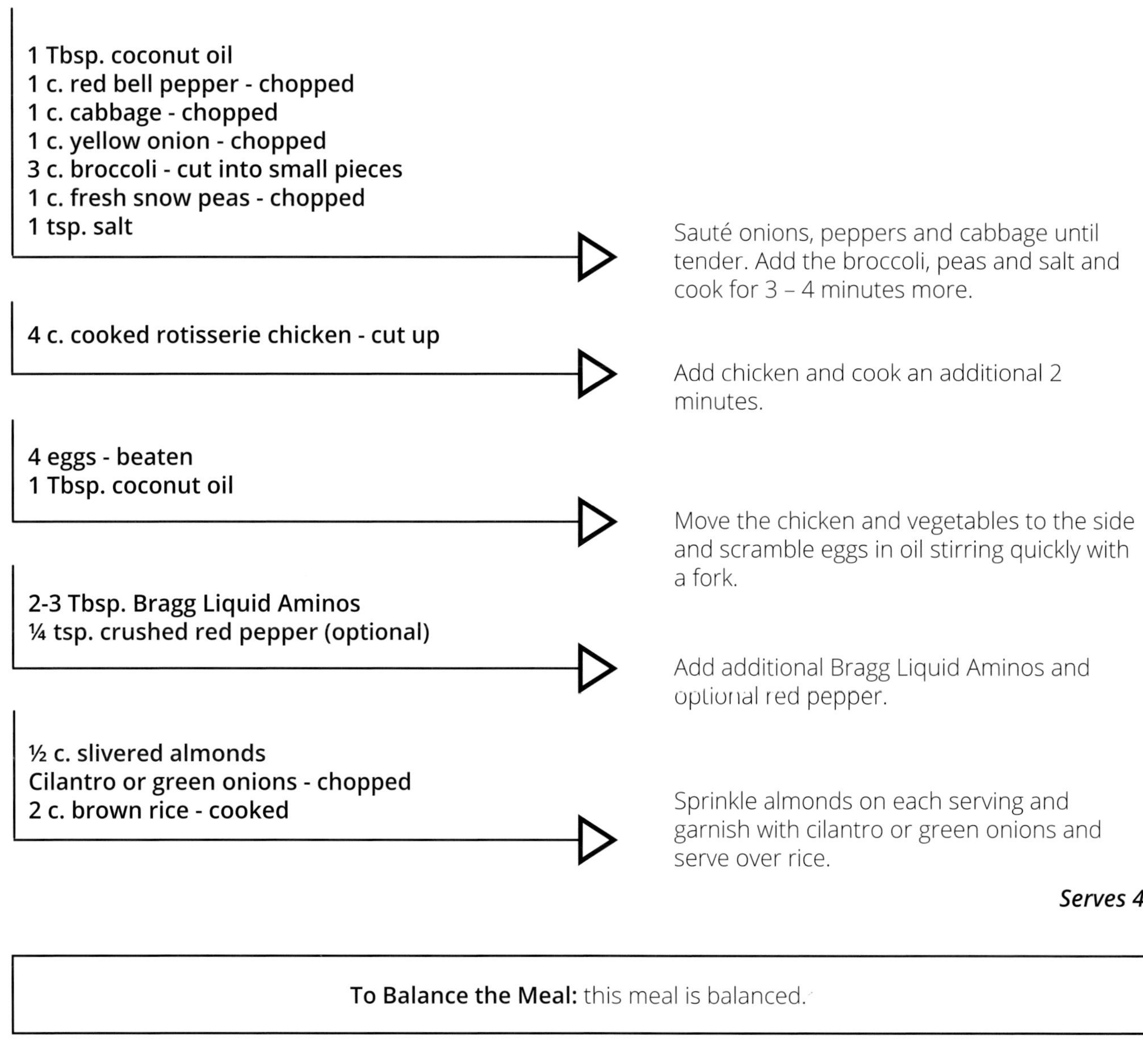

1 Tbsp. coconut oil
1 c. red bell pepper - chopped
1 c. cabbage - chopped
1 c. yellow onion - chopped
3 c. broccoli - cut into small pieces
1 c. fresh snow peas - chopped
1 tsp. salt

Sauté onions, peppers and cabbage until tender. Add the broccoli, peas and salt and cook for 3 – 4 minutes more.

4 c. cooked rotisserie chicken - cut up

Add chicken and cook an additional 2 minutes.

4 eggs - beaten
1 Tbsp. coconut oil

Move the chicken and vegetables to the side and scramble eggs in oil stirring quickly with a fork.

2-3 Tbsp. Bragg Liquid Aminos
¼ tsp. crushed red pepper (optional)

Add additional Bragg Liquid Aminos and optional red pepper.

½ c. slivered almonds
Cilantro or green onions - chopped
2 c. brown rice - cooked

Sprinkle almonds on each serving and garnish with cilantro or green onions and serve over rice.

Serves 4

To Balance the Meal: this meal is balanced.

To make gluten free:
This is gluten free

To make dairy free:
This is dairy free

Indian Curry

1 Tbsp. coconut oil
1½ lb. boneless/skinless chicken thighs - cut into 1" pieces

Melt coconut oil in a large skillet or Dutch oven. Brown chicken thighs on both sides. Remove and set aside.

2 tsp. coconut oil
2 cloves garlic - minced
1 Tbsp. curry powder
3 c. cauliflower - cut into bite-sized pieces
1 c. sweet potato - cut into small cubes
1 c. green beans - cut into bite-sized pieces

In the same pan, heat 2 tsp oil and add garlic and curry powder and cook for 1 minute, until fragrant. Add cauliflower, sweet potatoes and green beans and stir to mix.

½ c. chicken broth
½ can coconut milk
Cilantro or parsley (optional garnish)

Stir in chicken broth, coconut milk and reserved chicken and simmer on med-low for 25 - 30 minutes, until vegetables and chicken are cooked through.

Serves 4

To Balance the Meal: this meal is balanced.

To make gluten free:
This is gluten free

To make dairy free:
This is dairy free

Thai Chicken Curry

1 Tbsp. coconut oil
2 cloves garlic - minced
1 Tbsp. red curry paste (or to taste)
2 c. onions - chopped

In a large skillet or Dutch oven, heat coconut oil and add onions and cook for 3 – 4 minutes. Add the garlic and curry paste and stir until fragrant.

2 c. carrots - shredded
1 c. red peppers - chopped
1 c. green beans - cut into 1" pieces
2 c. spinach leaves - chopped
1 tsp. salt (or fish sauce)

Add the carrots, peppers and green beans and sauté for 3 minutes. Add spinach and cook until wilted. Season with salt.

4 c. cooked chicken (rotisserie) - cut up
½ c. chicken broth - organic/preservative free
1 can coconut milk
2 Tbsp. coconut aminos
Basil leaves/cilantro (optional)

Add chicken, broth, coconut milk and coconut aminos and simmer until vegetables are cooked through. Finish with torn basil leaves or chopped cilantro.

Serves 4

To Balance the Meal: serve over ½ c. cooked rice and garnish with lime wedges and fresh cilantro, if desired.

To make gluten free:
This is gluten free

To make dairy free:
This is dairy free

The Weight & Wellness Way to Reduce Pain and Inflammation

Every day I suffer from aches and pains. Will this eating plan offer me any help?

By changing the way you eat, you can reduce or even eliminate many of your aches and pains. At Nutritional Weight & Wellness, we teach that sugar and processed carbohydrates contribute to generalized inflammation and even to painful joints and muscles. Replace processed foods, such as canned soups, cereal and cookies with vegetables, beneficial fats and protein and see how much better you feel. It has worked like magic for many of our clients.

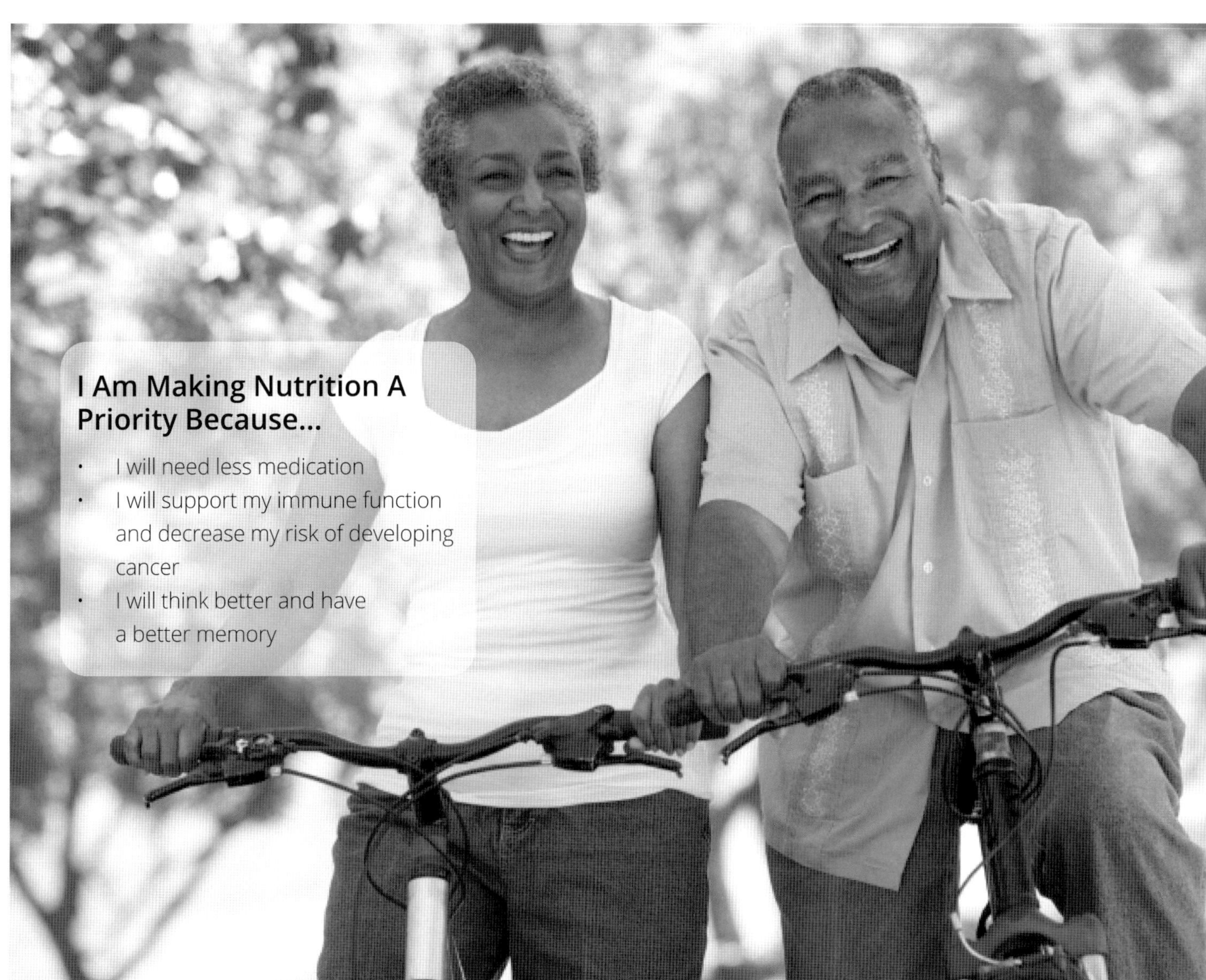

I Am Making Nutrition A Priority Because...

- I will need less medication
- I will support my immune function and decrease my risk of developing cancer
- I will think better and have a better memory

Apple Cinnamon Pork Roast

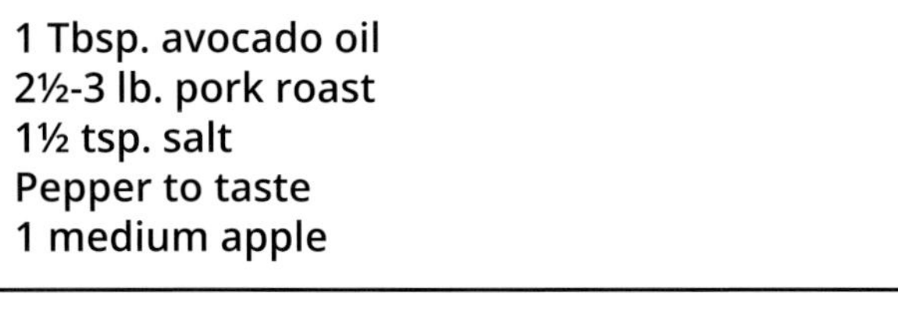

1 Tbsp. avocado oil
2½-3 lb. pork roast
1½ tsp. salt
Pepper to taste
1 medium apple

Season the pork with salt and pepper. Heat avocado oil in a large skillet over med-high heat and brown the roast on all sides. Core and very thinly slice the apple. Cut slits into roast on all sides. Insert apple slices into slits.

2 tsp. chili powder
1 Tbsp. cinnamon
2 Tbsp. apple cider vinegar
1 medium onion - sliced
1 c. chicken stock

Transfer roast to a slow cooker and sprinkle with cinnamon and chili powder. Pour in vinegar and stock and scatter onion slices around the roast. Cook on low for 6-8 hours.

Serves 8

To Balance the Meal: serve with 1 c. roasted Brussels sprouts, ½ c. carrots and 2 tsp. butter.

To make gluten free:
This is gluten free

To make dairy free:
This is dairy free

Dijon Crockpot® Pork Chops

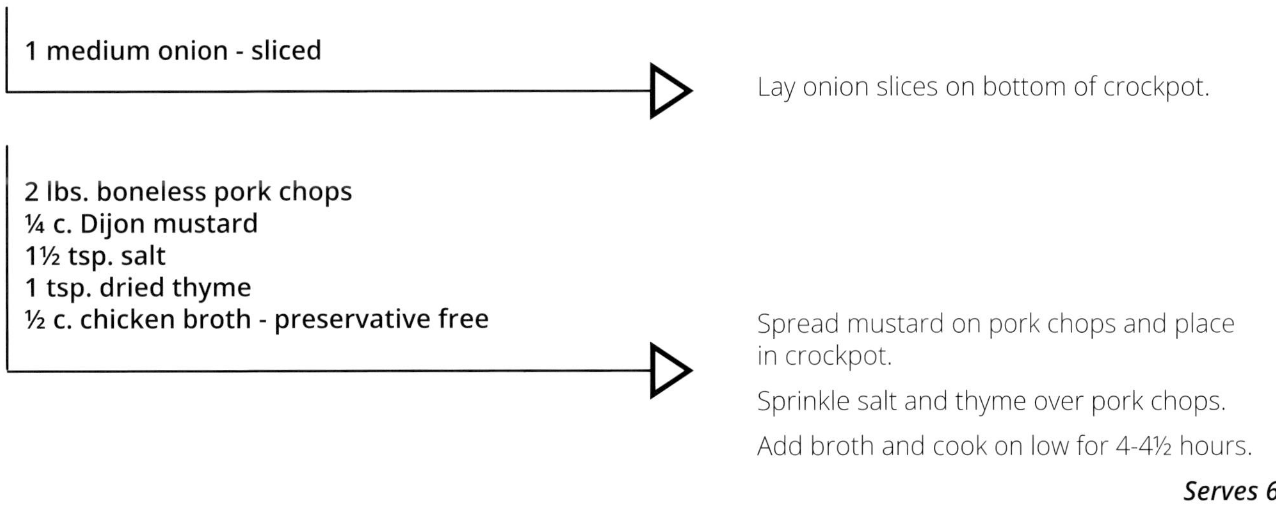

1 medium onion - sliced

Lay onion slices on bottom of crockpot.

2 lbs. boneless pork chops
¼ c. Dijon mustard
1½ tsp. salt
1 tsp. dried thyme
½ c. chicken broth - preservative free

Spread mustard on pork chops and place in crockpot.

Sprinkle salt and thyme over pork chops.

Add broth and cook on low for 4-4½ hours.

Serves 6

To Balance the Meal: serve with 2 c. sautéed cabbage, ½ c. cooked carrots and 2 tsp. butter.

To make gluten free:
This is gluten free

To make dairy free:
Substitute coconut oil for butter

Instant Pot Citrus Pork

1 Tbsp. kosher salt
2 tsp. garlic powder
Zest of 1 orange
Zest of 1 lime
1 tsp. ground black pepper
5 lbs. boneless pork shoulder - cut into 3-4 pieces

In a small bowl, mix salt, garlic, orange zest, lime zest and pepper. Season pork pieces with spice mixture.

1 Tbsp. coconut oil or ghee
½ c. liquid (including citrus juice from orange and lime plus water if needed)

Select Instant Pot SAUTE function; heat coconut oil. Sear pork in batches, until well browned on the outside.

Add liquid and return meat to the pot. Twist lid to seal.

Select MANUAL function and set timer for 70 minutes. Allow to naturally depressurize.

For a slow cooker, the searing step can either be skipped (omit the coconut oil/ghee) or done in a pan and transferred to the slow cooker. Cook about 6-8 hours on low or until tender enough to shred.

Serves 12

To Balance the Meal: serve with ½ c. potato, 2 c. green beans and 2 tsp. butter.

To make gluten free:
This meal is gluten free

To make dairy free:
Substitute coconut or avocado oil for butter

Lamb Chops with Lemon

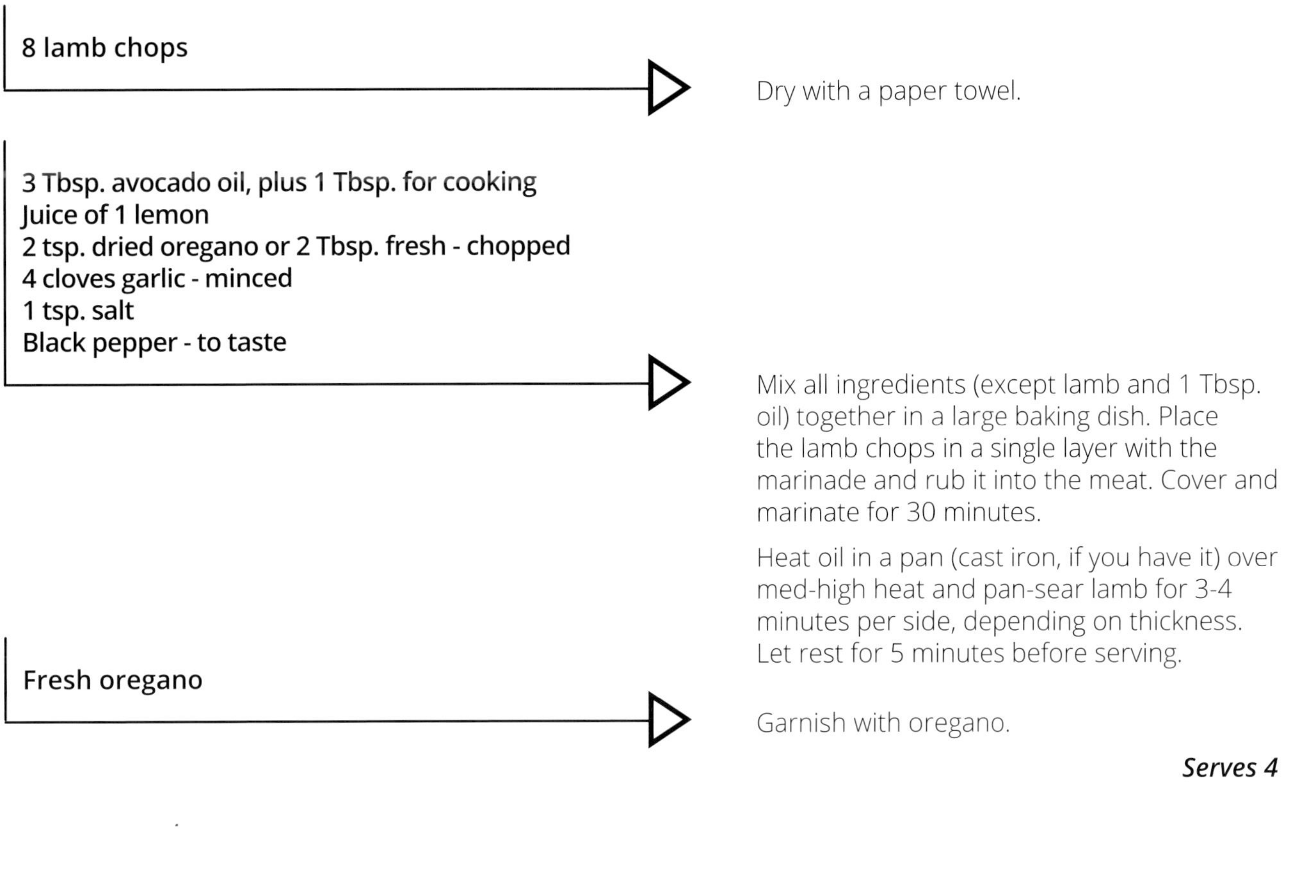

8 lamb chops

Dry with a paper towel.

3 Tbsp. avocado oil, plus 1 Tbsp. for cooking
Juice of 1 lemon
2 tsp. dried oregano or 2 Tbsp. fresh - chopped
4 cloves garlic - minced
1 tsp. salt
Black pepper - to taste

Mix all ingredients (except lamb and 1 Tbsp. oil) together in a large baking dish. Place the lamb chops in a single layer with the marinade and rub it into the meat. Cover and marinate for 30 minutes.

Heat oil in a pan (cast iron, if you have it) over med-high heat and pan-sear lamb for 3-4 minutes per side, depending on thickness. Let rest for 5 minutes before serving.

Fresh oregano

Garnish with oregano.

Serves 4

To Balance the Meal: Serve with 2 c. of sauteed spinach or chard, drizzled with 1 Tbsp. olive oil and ½ c. Sweet Potato Wedges (p. 155).

To make gluten free:
This is gluten free

To make dairy free:
This is dairy free

The Weight & Wellness Way to Better Moods

Will this plan help me manage my depression?

Research has found that the cause of depression is biochemical. As nutritionists, we know that when people consistently balance their meals with animal protein, vegetable carbohydrates and good fats, they are more focused, energetic and optimistic. Sadly, balanced eating is often one of the first things we abandon when our mood is low or we are depressed, which in turn contributes to more low moods and depression. Researchers have found that the brain chemicals serotonin and dopamine determine happiness, self-esteem and energy levels. These and other brain chemicals require adequate animal protein, essential fatty acids (especially the Omega-3s) and healthy fats. Nutritional Weight & Wellness clients report that eating the Weight & Wellness Way lifts their moods, energy and sense of well-being.

Timm's success story—depression managed with real food

Ever since I can remember, I have experienced depression and problems with addiction; first to alcohol, then to drugs and sugar. I wasn't able to run my business because I couldn't get off the couch and get to work. That was when my wife decided I needed to do something. Medications didn't seem to help me much. With my wife's encouragement, I decided to look at food as my antidepressant. I am happy to say that by carefully balancing my eating with sufficient protein, lots of veggies and good fats, I am positive and productive. I recognize that I need to be very careful about my foods. I need to eat on schedule. I carry healthy food with me at all times—even on job sites, because fast food will make me depressed. Is this careful way of eating worth it? I can only say that it has saved my life, my marriage and my business.

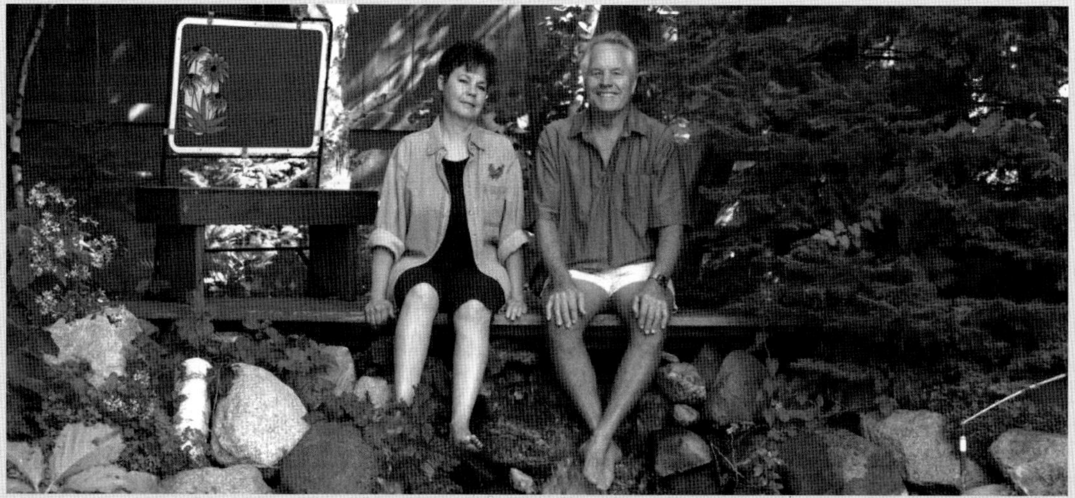

Timm feeling healthy and happy with his wife Oralee

Confetti Turkey Loaf

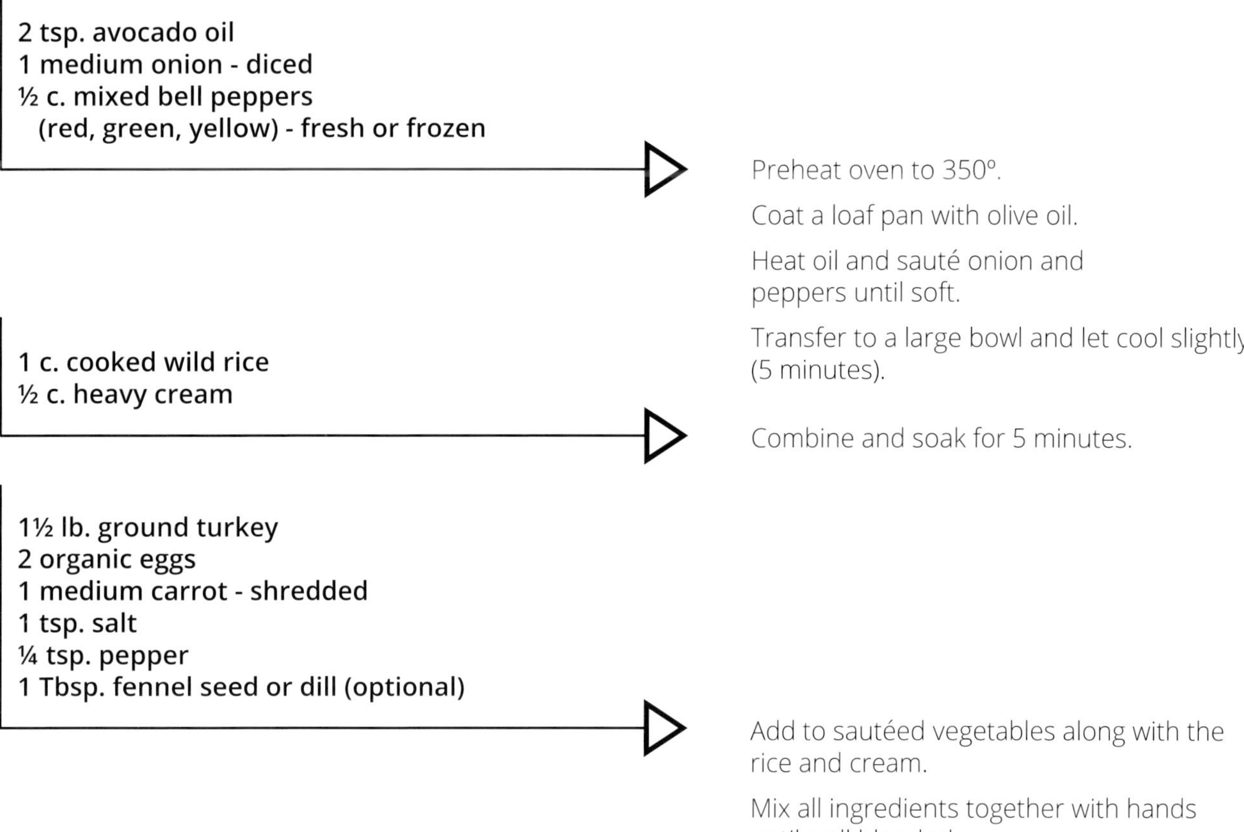

2 tsp. avocado oil
1 medium onion - diced
½ c. mixed bell peppers
(red, green, yellow) - fresh or frozen

Preheat oven to 350º.

Coat a loaf pan with olive oil.

Heat oil and sauté onion and peppers until soft.

Transfer to a large bowl and let cool slightly (5 minutes).

1 c. cooked wild rice
½ c. heavy cream

Combine and soak for 5 minutes.

1½ lb. ground turkey
2 organic eggs
1 medium carrot - shredded
1 tsp. salt
¼ tsp. pepper
1 Tbsp. fennel seed or dill (optional)

Add to sautéed vegetables along with the rice and cream.

Mix all ingredients together with hands until well blended.

Shape the meat into the loaf pan and bake at 350º for 1 hour.

Serves 6

To Balance the Meal: serve with 1 c. steamed vegetables and 1 c. hot spaghetti squash, tossed with 1 Tbsp. butter and fresh basil or parsley.

To make gluten free:
This meal is gluten free

To make dairy free:
Use coconut milk instead of cream and coconut oil instead of butter

Indian-Style Turkey Cutlet

Juice and zest from 1 lime
1 c. plain full-fat yogurt
1 Tbsp. avocado oil
2 tsp. grated ginger
1 tsp. ground cumin
1 tsp. ground coriander
1 tsp. salt
1 clove garlic

Preheat grill to medium

In large bowl, mix, lime juice, yogurt, avocado oil, ginger, cumin, coriander, salt, and garlic until blended.

1 lb. turkey cutlets
Cilantro sprigs
Lime wedges

Just before grilling, add turkey cutlets to bowl with yogurt mixture, stirring to coat cutlets. (Do not let cutlets marinate in mixture.) Place turkey on grill and cook for 3 minutes per side, until they are cooked through. Serve with lime wedges. Garnish with cilantro.

Serves 4

To Balance the Meal: serve with ½ c. brown rice and 1 c. steamed cauliflower with 1 Tbsp. butter.

To make gluten free:
This meal is gluten free

To make dairy free:
Use full-fat coconut milk instead of yogurt.

Italian-Style Turkey Steaks

2 Tbsp. avocado or coconut oil
1¼ lb. turkey breast - sliced into 1" slices
1 c. mushrooms - sliced

Brown the turkey and mushrooms in a skillet on both sides.

Juice and zest of 2 lemons
½ c. chicken broth - preservative free
1 c. tomatoes - chopped
2 Tbsp. capers
1 c. fresh spinach - chopped
¼ c. fresh parsley - chopped
Salt and pepper to taste

Add all except spinach and parsley to skillet and bring to a boil.

Reduce heat, cover, add spinach and cook until turkey is tender (about 6-8 minutes). Garnish with parsley.

Serves 4

To Balance the Meal: serve with ½ c. cannellini beans drizzled with 1 Tbsp. olive oil and 2 c. mixed steamed vegetables with 1 tsp. olive oil.

To make gluten free:
This meal is gluten free

To make dairy free:
This meal is dairy free

Lemon Baked Turkey Breast

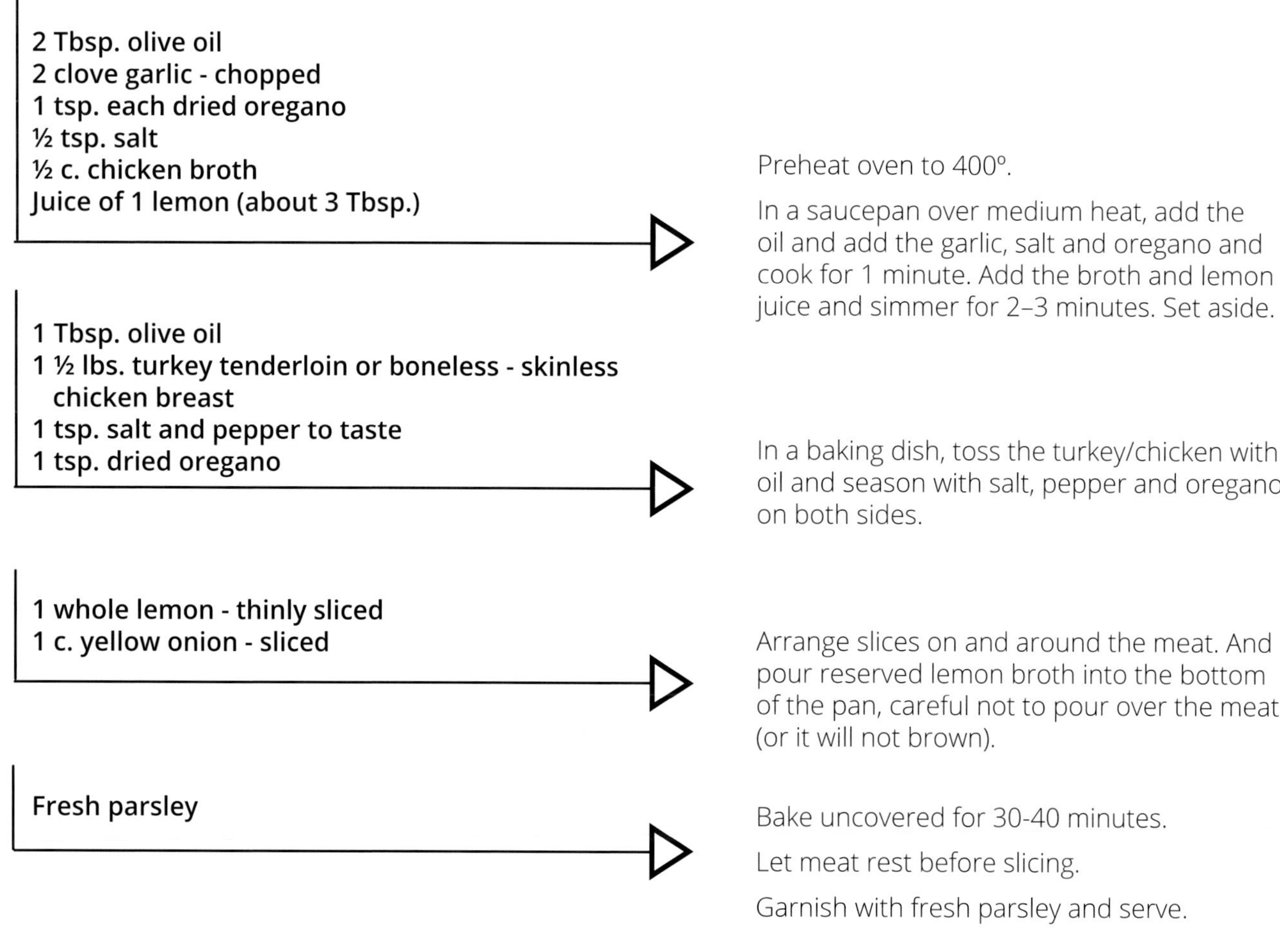

2 Tbsp. olive oil
2 clove garlic - chopped
1 tsp. each dried oregano
½ tsp. salt
½ c. chicken broth
Juice of 1 lemon (about 3 Tbsp.)

Preheat oven to 400°.

In a saucepan over medium heat, add the oil and add the garlic, salt and oregano and cook for 1 minute. Add the broth and lemon juice and simmer for 2–3 minutes. Set aside.

1 Tbsp. olive oil
1 ½ lbs. turkey tenderloin or boneless - skinless chicken breast
1 tsp. salt and pepper to taste
1 tsp. dried oregano

In a baking dish, toss the turkey/chicken with oil and season with salt, pepper and oregano on both sides.

1 whole lemon - thinly sliced
1 c. yellow onion - sliced

Arrange slices on and around the meat. And pour reserved lemon broth into the bottom of the pan, careful not to pour over the meat (or it will not brown).

Fresh parsley

Bake uncovered for 30-40 minutes.

Let meat rest before slicing.

Garnish with fresh parsley and serve.

Serves 4

To Balance the Meal: 2 c. cooked green beans and ¾ c. Mashed Potatoes and Cauliflower (p. 145). Use 1 tsp. butter on vegetables.

To make gluten free:
This meal is gluten free

To make dairy free:
Use coconut oil instead of butter

Minnesota Turkey and Wild Rice Casserole

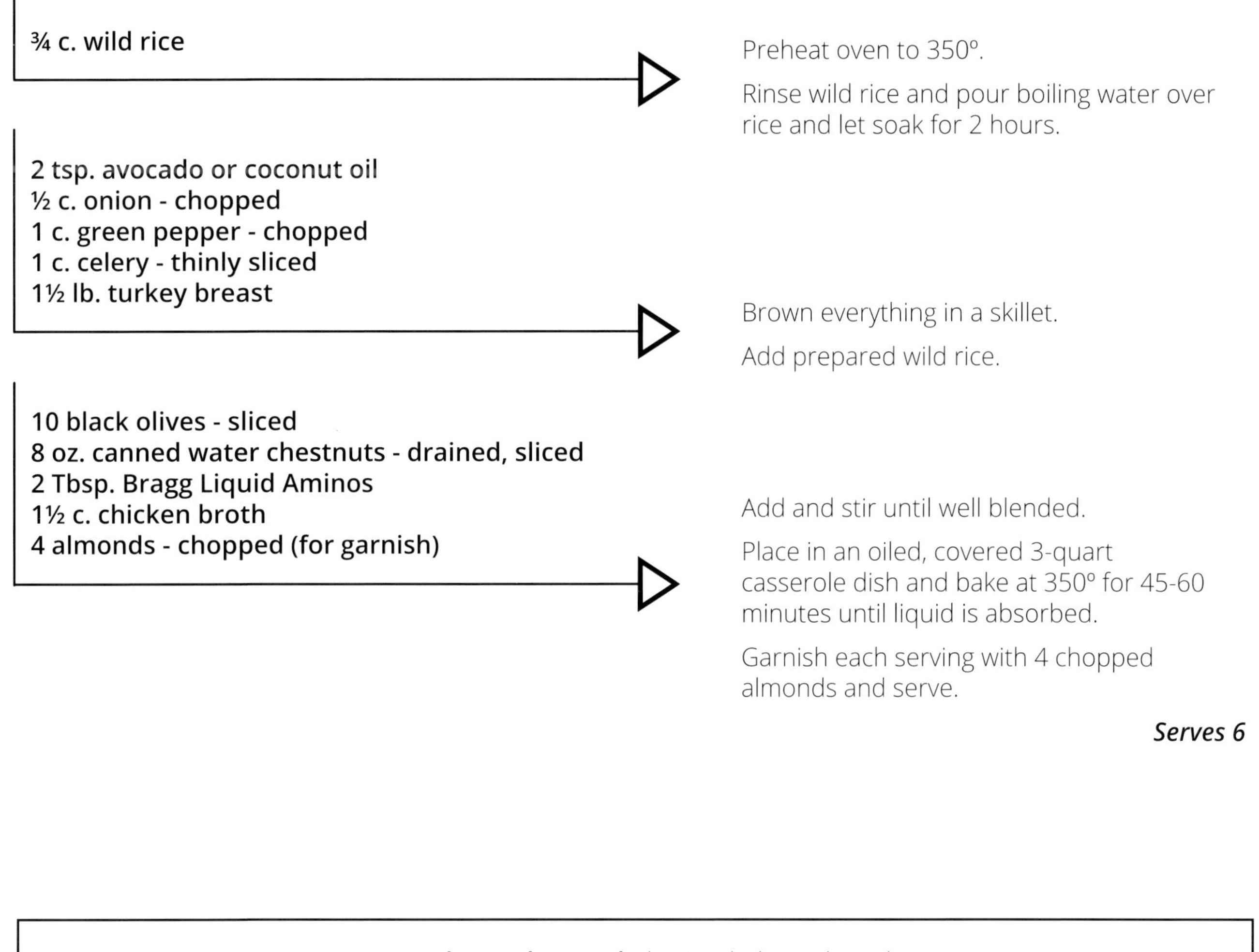

Preheat oven to 350º.

Rinse wild rice and pour boiling water over rice and let soak for 2 hours.

Brown everything in a skillet.

Add prepared wild rice.

Add and stir until well blended.

Place in an oiled, covered 3-quart casserole dish and bake at 350º for 45-60 minutes until liquid is absorbed.

Garnish each serving with 4 chopped almonds and serve.

Serves 6

To Balance the Meal: this is a balanced meal.

To make gluten free:
This meal is gluten free

To make dairy free:
This meal is dairy free

Mustard Baked Turkey Cutlet

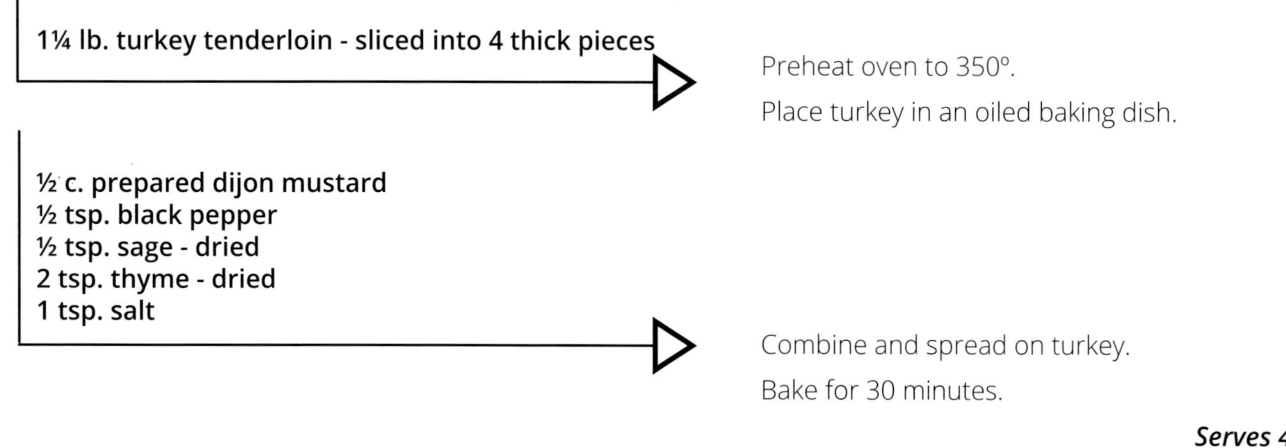

1¼ lb. turkey tenderloin - sliced into 4 thick pieces

Preheat oven to 350°.
Place turkey in an oiled baking dish.

½ c. prepared dijon mustard
½ tsp. black pepper
½ tsp. sage - dried
2 tsp. thyme - dried
1 tsp. salt

Combine and spread on turkey.
Bake for 30 minutes.

Serves 4

To Balance the Meal: serve with 2 c. raw vegetable sticks (celery, cucumber, zucchini, carrots, etc.) and 2 Tbsp. Super Simple Ranch Dressing for dip (p. 135).

To make gluten free:
This meal is gluten free

To make dairy free:
Use dairy-free dressing

Southwestern Shepherd's Pie

Topping
2 lbs. sweet potatoes - peeled and diced
¼ c. coconut milk or heavy cream
2 Tbsp. butter (or olive oil)
1 tsp. salt
¼ c. fresh herbs - finely chopped (cilantro, parsley)

In a 4 qt. saucepan, heat 1 cup of water (or bone broth) and 1 tsp salt.

Add the sweet potatoes and steam, covered for 25 - 30 minutes. (make filling while this cooks)

Finish with the butter/oil and coconut milk and mash – add fresh herbs, if using.

Set aside.

Filling
2 Tbsp. avocado oil (ghee, lard or bacon fat), divided
2 lbs. ground turkey (preferably dark meat)
½ tsp. smoked chipotle pepper or chili powder
1 tsp. ground cumin
1 ½ tsp. salt and pepper to taste
2 Tbsp. tomato paste
¼-1/3 c. chicken stock (or bone broth)
3 c. chopped onion
3 c. chopped red/yellow peppers
1, 10-oz. bag of riced cauliflower (fresh or frozen)
2-4 cloves of garlic - minced

Preheat oven to 400º.

This can be made in a large oven-proof skillet or in a 9 x 13" pan.

Heat large sauté pan and add 1 Tbsp oil until shimmering. Add the ground turkey and ½ tsp salt. As it browns, tilt the pan and spoon off the water (turkey can have up to 6% water).

Add the cumin and chili powder – then the tomato paste and stir until fragrant. Remove meat from pan and set aside.

In same pan, add 1 Tbsp oil and add the onions and peppers – cook until onions are translucent. Add the garlic and cook for 1 minute more.

Add the cauliflower, stock and 1 tsp salt –(if using frozen, cook until thawed).

Return the meat to the pan or transfer meat and vegetables to a baking dish and mix well; check seasonings.

Top with the mashed potatoes. Using a spatula create a smooth even coating and bake in the oven for 25 minutes.

Serves 6

To Balance the Meal: this is a balanced meal.

To make gluten free:
This is gluten free

To make dairy free:
Use coconut milk and olive oil in place of cream and butter

Turkey or Chicken Nuggets

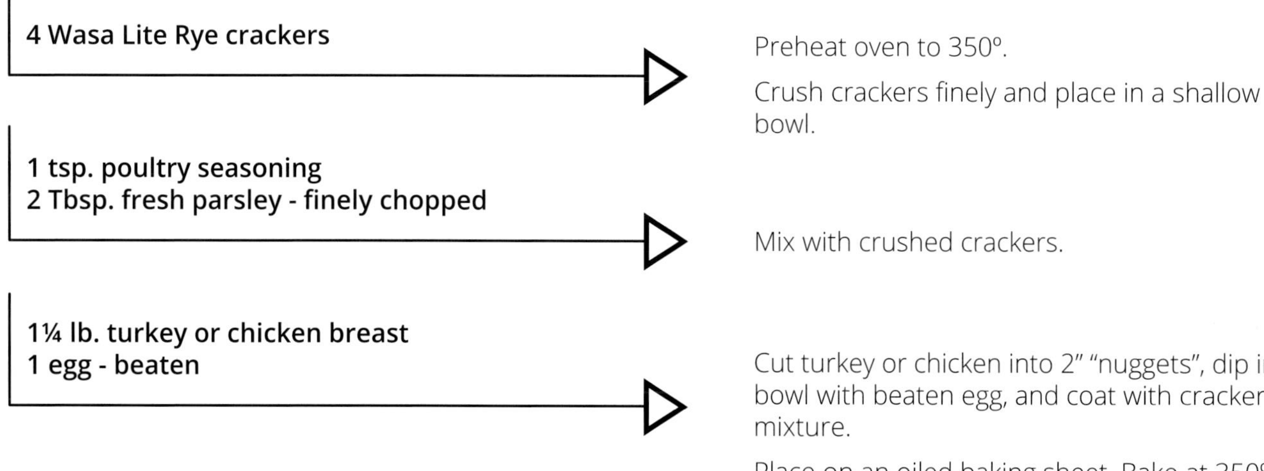

4 Wasa Lite Rye crackers

Preheat oven to 350°.

Crush crackers finely and place in a shallow bowl.

1 tsp. poultry seasoning
2 Tbsp. fresh parsley - finely chopped

Mix with crushed crackers.

1¼ lb. turkey or chicken breast
1 egg - beaten

Cut turkey or chicken into 2" "nuggets", dip in bowl with beaten egg, and coat with cracker mixture.

Place on an oiled baking sheet. Bake at 350° for 30 minutes, turning once.

Serves 4

To Balance the Meal: serve with 1 c. fresh cut vegetables and 2 Tbsp. Super Simple Ranch Dressing (p. 135)

To make gluten free:
Substitute almond meal for Wasa crackers

To make dairy free:
Use a dairy-free dressing

Turkey Quinoa Stew

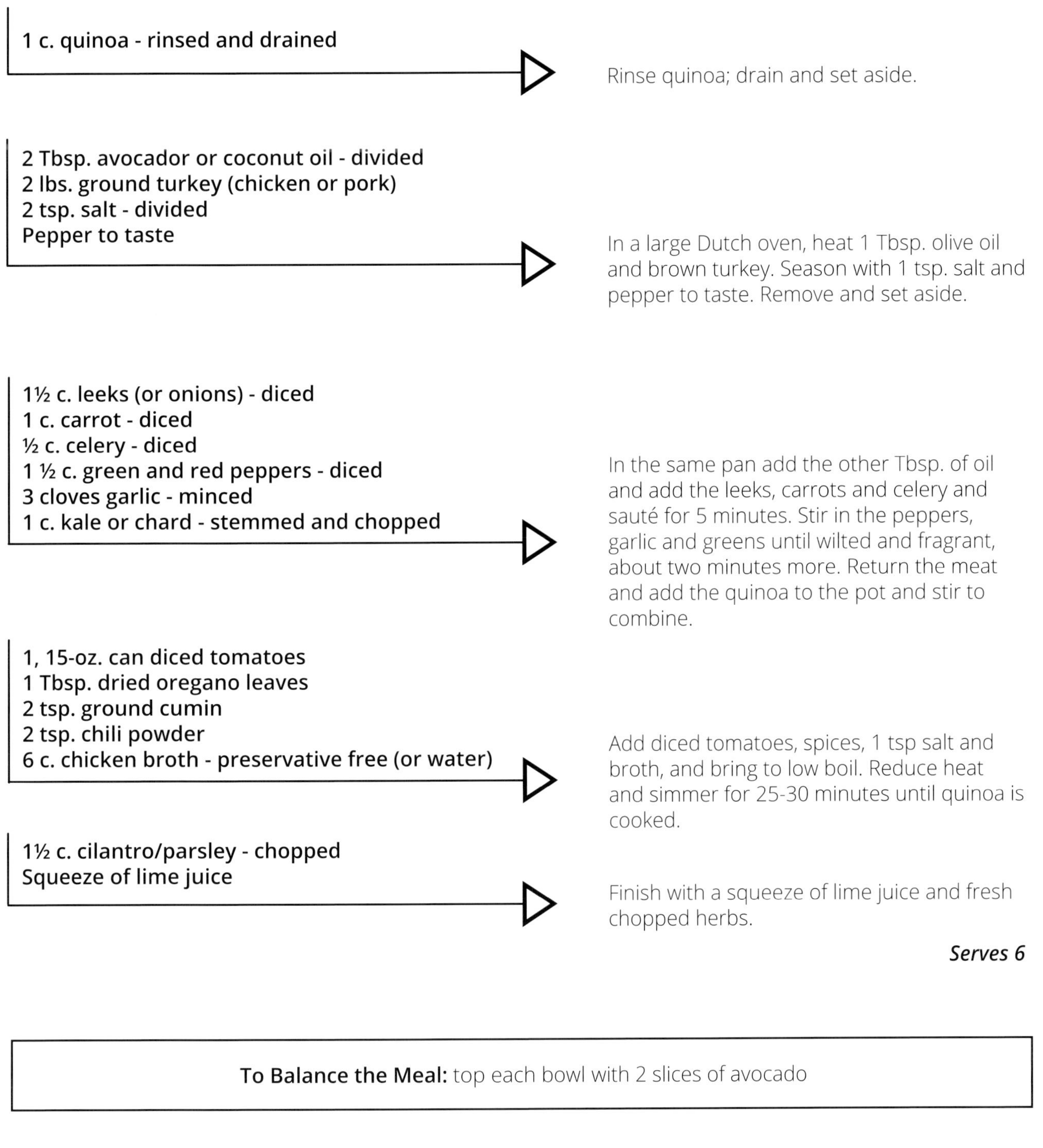

1 c. quinoa - rinsed and drained

Rinse quinoa; drain and set aside.

2 Tbsp. avocador or coconut oil - divided
2 lbs. ground turkey (chicken or pork)
2 tsp. salt - divided
Pepper to taste

In a large Dutch oven, heat 1 Tbsp. olive oil and brown turkey. Season with 1 tsp. salt and pepper to taste. Remove and set aside.

1½ c. leeks (or onions) - diced
1 c. carrot - diced
½ c. celery - diced
1 ½ c. green and red peppers - diced
3 cloves garlic - minced
1 c. kale or chard - stemmed and chopped

In the same pan add the other Tbsp. of oil and add the leeks, carrots and celery and sauté for 5 minutes. Stir in the peppers, garlic and greens until wilted and fragrant, about two minutes more. Return the meat and add the quinoa to the pot and stir to combine.

1, 15-oz. can diced tomatoes
1 Tbsp. dried oregano leaves
2 tsp. ground cumin
2 tsp. chili powder
6 c. chicken broth - preservative free (or water)

Add diced tomatoes, spices, 1 tsp salt and broth, and bring to low boil. Reduce heat and simmer for 25-30 minutes until quinoa is cooked.

1½ c. cilantro/parsley - chopped
Squeeze of lime juice

Finish with a squeeze of lime juice and fresh chopped herbs.

Serves 6

To Balance the Meal: top each bowl with 2 slices of avocado

To make gluten free:
This meal is gluten free

To make dairy free:
This meal is dairy free

Turkey and Vegetables Meal-in-a-Bag

½ c. onion - diced
½ c. red bell pepper - chopped
2 tsp. balsamic vinegar
1 clove garlic - minced
1 tsp. salt
1 tsp. cumin
2 Tbsp. coconut oil

Preheat oven to 350°.

Sauté vegetables in coconut oil, add seasonings.

2 lb. ground turkey

In a bowl, combine turkey with sautéed vegetables. Shape into 6 patties and place in individual parchment bags*.

1½ c. small potato - sliced
1½ c. carrots - sliced
½ c. leek - sliced
6 c. cauliflower - cut into bite-size pieces
6 c. broccoli - cut into bite-size pieces
4 Tbsp. Bragg Liquid Aminos
2 Tbsp. olive oil

Combine vegetables and add olive oil, Bragg Liquid Aminos, and salt mixture. Divide vegetables evenly in 6 parchment bags and place on a baking sheet.

Bake at 350° for 40-45 minutes.

Serves 6

To Balance the Meal: this meal is balanced.

To make gluten free:
This is gluten free

To make dairy free:
This is dairy free

** Can use a parchment sheet folded over and creased to seal.*

The Weight & Wellness Way:
The Answer to Your Digestive Problems

I have serious digestive problems, and I'm afraid to eat vegetables because they give me gas and diarrhea.

What might be causing your digestive problems?

- Processed foods
- Foods containing sugar and high fructose corn syrup
- Soda
- Artificial sweeteners in soda, mints and gum
- Food sensitivities to gluten or dairy
- Overuse of antibiotics
- Overuse of anti-inflammatory medications
- Lack of beneficial bacteria

Many people experience fewer symptoms just by following the Weight & Wellness eating plan. Others benefit from additional information and services. You may want to consider an individual nutrition consultation or taking one of the following classes:

- Gut Reaction: Restore Digestive Health through Nutrition
- Going Gluten Free the Healthy Way

Lee's success story—regular again and worry-free

Lee entered the doors of Nutritional Weight & Wellness in July of 2011. Lee had suffered for many years with diarrhea and not just occasional bouts of it; this was a chronic problem for her. It was maddening. She visited several doctors over the years to try and solve the problem, but no underlying conditions were ever identified. She went through multiple colonoscopies and had fecal samples tested to figure out the problem. Time after time, her doctors came back to her with no diagnosis and no solution. Doctors recommended that she continue her use of Imodium® to manage the problem.

Lee

Referred by a friend to Nutritional Weight & Wellness, Lee went as a last resort for solving her chronic diarrhea. Lee had tried so many other things, but was willing to give nutrition a try. She made an appointment with Darlene Kvist, and Darlene started by eliminating dairy and gluten from Lee's diet. ***Lee saw immediate results and was able to stop taking her Imodium®.*** *When her problem crept up again, Lee met with Darlene to further refine her diet and has had normal bowel movements since that time.* ***She is now able to enjoy a wide variety of foods, including some dairy again, and doesn't worry any longer about having diarrhea.***

"Darlene is amazing, I would recommend her to anyone" remarked Lee. "I also lost 10 pounds along the way—which was not something I was looking to do." *Lee is happy to report that she recently enjoyed a vacation in London and felt wonderful the entire time.*

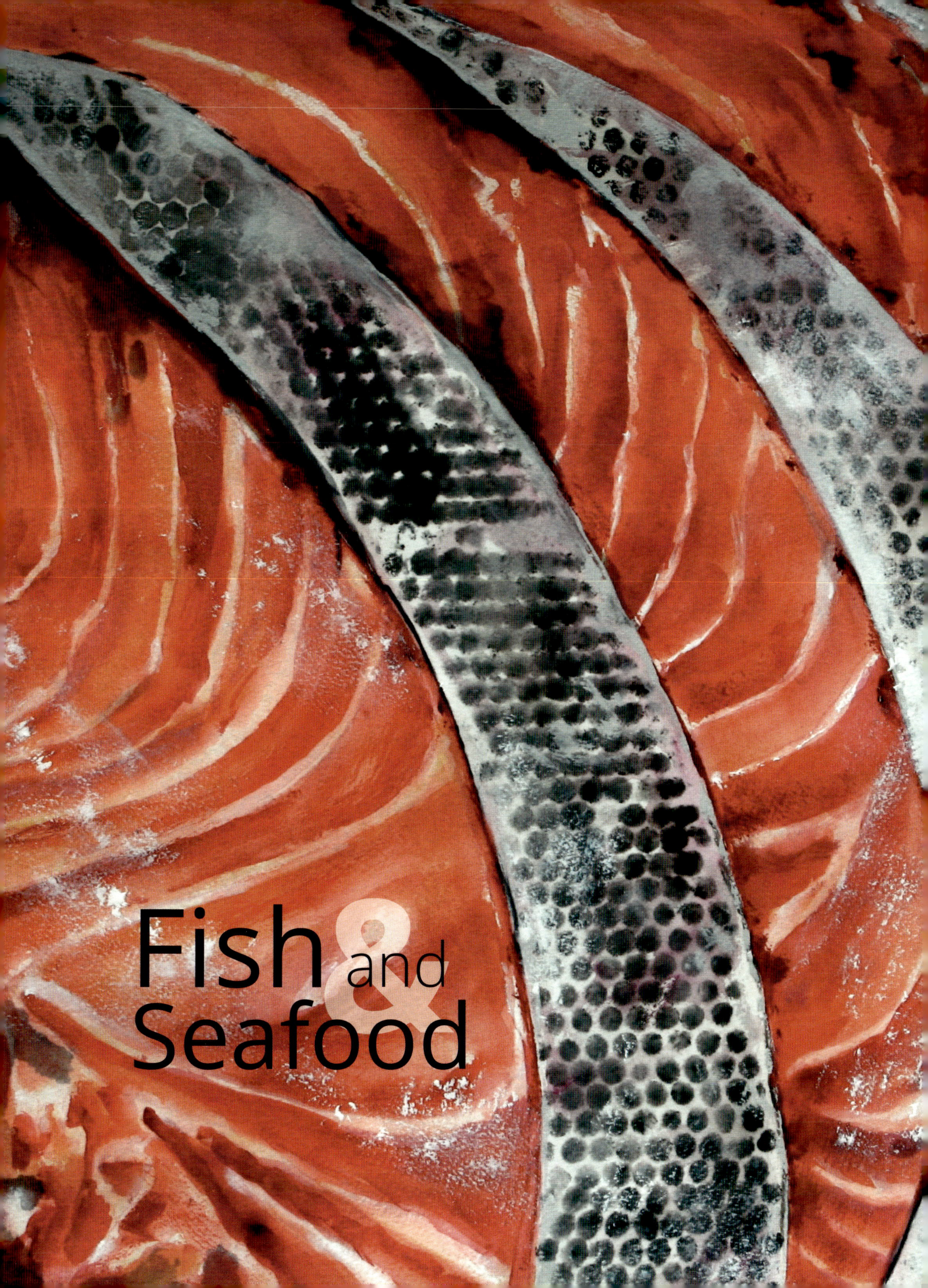

Fish & and Seafood

Baked Fish with Herbs

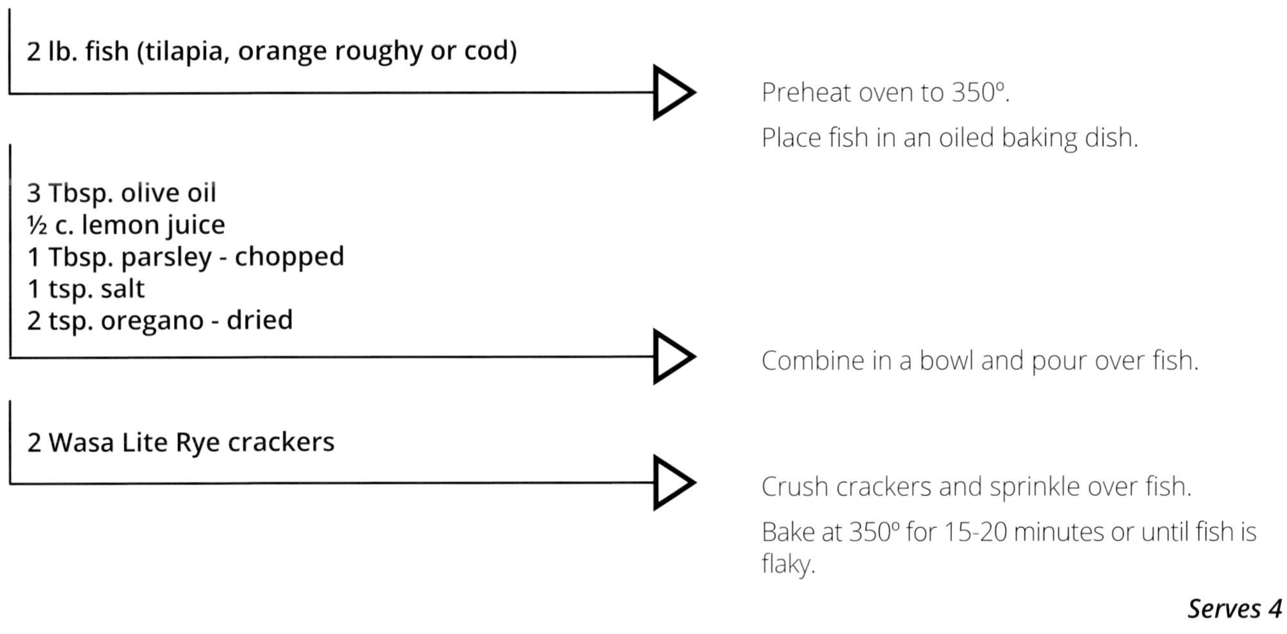

2 lb. fish (tilapia, orange roughy or cod)

Preheat oven to 350º.

Place fish in an oiled baking dish.

3 Tbsp. olive oil
½ c. lemon juice
1 Tbsp. parsley - chopped
1 tsp. salt
2 tsp. oregano - dried

Combine in a bowl and pour over fish.

2 Wasa Lite Rye crackers

Crush crackers and sprinkle over fish.

Bake at 350º for 15-20 minutes or until fish is flaky.

Serves 4

To Balance the Meal: serve with ½ c. quinoa, 12 asparagus spears and 2 tsp. butter.

To make gluten free:
Use almond meal instead of crackers

To make dairy free:
Use coconut oil instead of butter

Cajun Fish Fillets

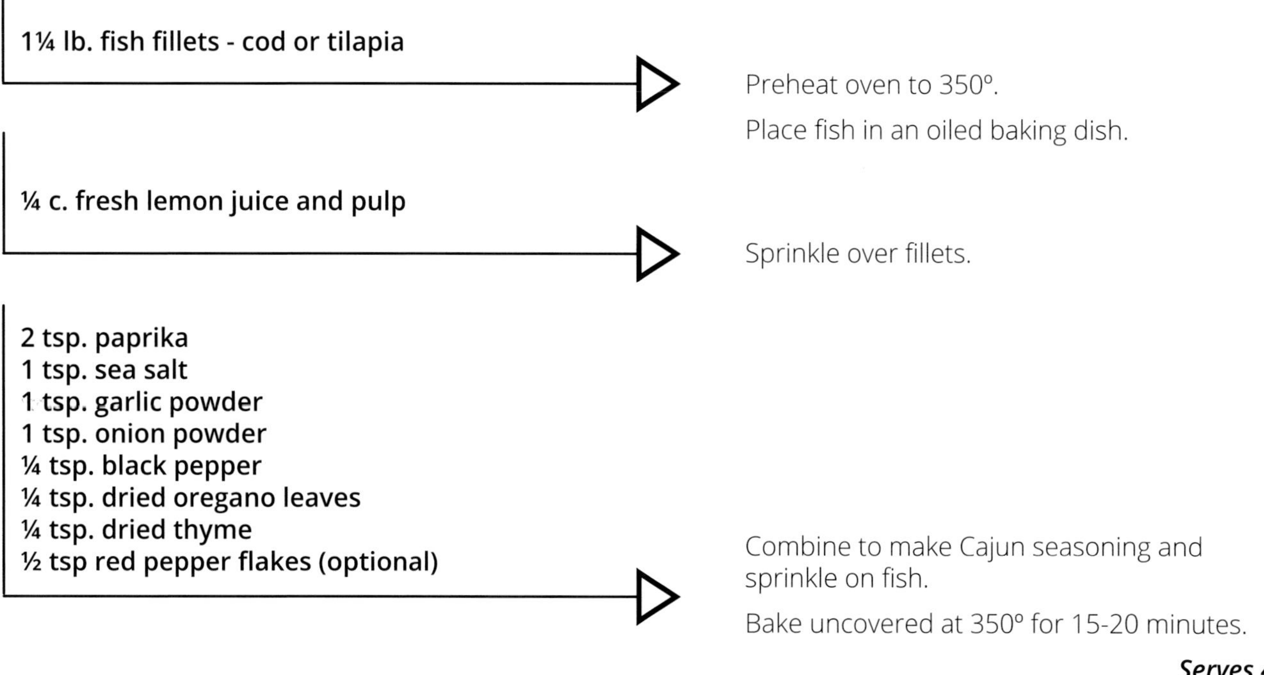

1¼ lb. fish fillets - cod or tilapia

Preheat oven to 350°.

Place fish in an oiled baking dish.

¼ c. fresh lemon juice and pulp

Sprinkle over fillets.

2 tsp. paprika
1 tsp. sea salt
1 tsp. garlic powder
1 tsp. onion powder
¼ tsp. black pepper
¼ tsp. dried oregano leaves
¼ tsp. dried thyme
½ tsp red pepper flakes (optional)

Combine to make Cajun seasoning and sprinkle on fish.

Bake uncovered at 350° for 15-20 minutes.

Serves 4

To Balance the Meal: serve with ½ ear of corn on the cob with 1 tsp. butter and ½ c. cooked Collard Greens (p. 142).

To make gluten free:
This meal is gluten free

To make dairy free:
Use coconut oil instead of butter

Cod with Peppers

½ yellow onion
4, 6-oz. skinless, boneless cod (halibut, tilapia) fillets
1½ tsp. salt, divided
Freshly ground black pepper
2 Tbsp. extra-virgin olive oil
1 lime

Preheat oven to 300°.

Thinly slice the onion and place in a medium baking dish. Place cod fillets on top of onion slices. Generously sprinkle fillets on both sides with 1 tsp. salt and season with black pepper. Drizzle 1 Tbsp. olive oil over, then finely grate zest from 1 lime on top; set lime aside. Turn fillets to coat. Prepare remaining ingredients.

4 garlic cloves - minced
1-2" piece ginger - grated
1 Tbsp. fresh thyme leaves - chopped, or 1 tsp. dried thyme
1 small bunch cilantro (or parsley) - chopped
1/3 c. scallions - chopped
1 red bell pepper - diced
½ jalapeno pepper - finely diced (optional)

Place garlic and ginger in a small bowl and add the remaining ingredients (including ½ tsp. salt) and toss to combine. Spoon mixture evenly over cod to completely cover. Bake until fish is opaque and cooked through and peppers are softened, 18 - 20 minutes.

Serves 4

To Balance the Meal: serve with 2 c. of Zucchini Sauté (p.156) and ½ c. roasted red potato topped with 1 Tbsp. butter.

To make gluten free:
This meal is gluten free

To make dairy free:
Substitute coconut oil for butter

Easy Fish and Vegetables

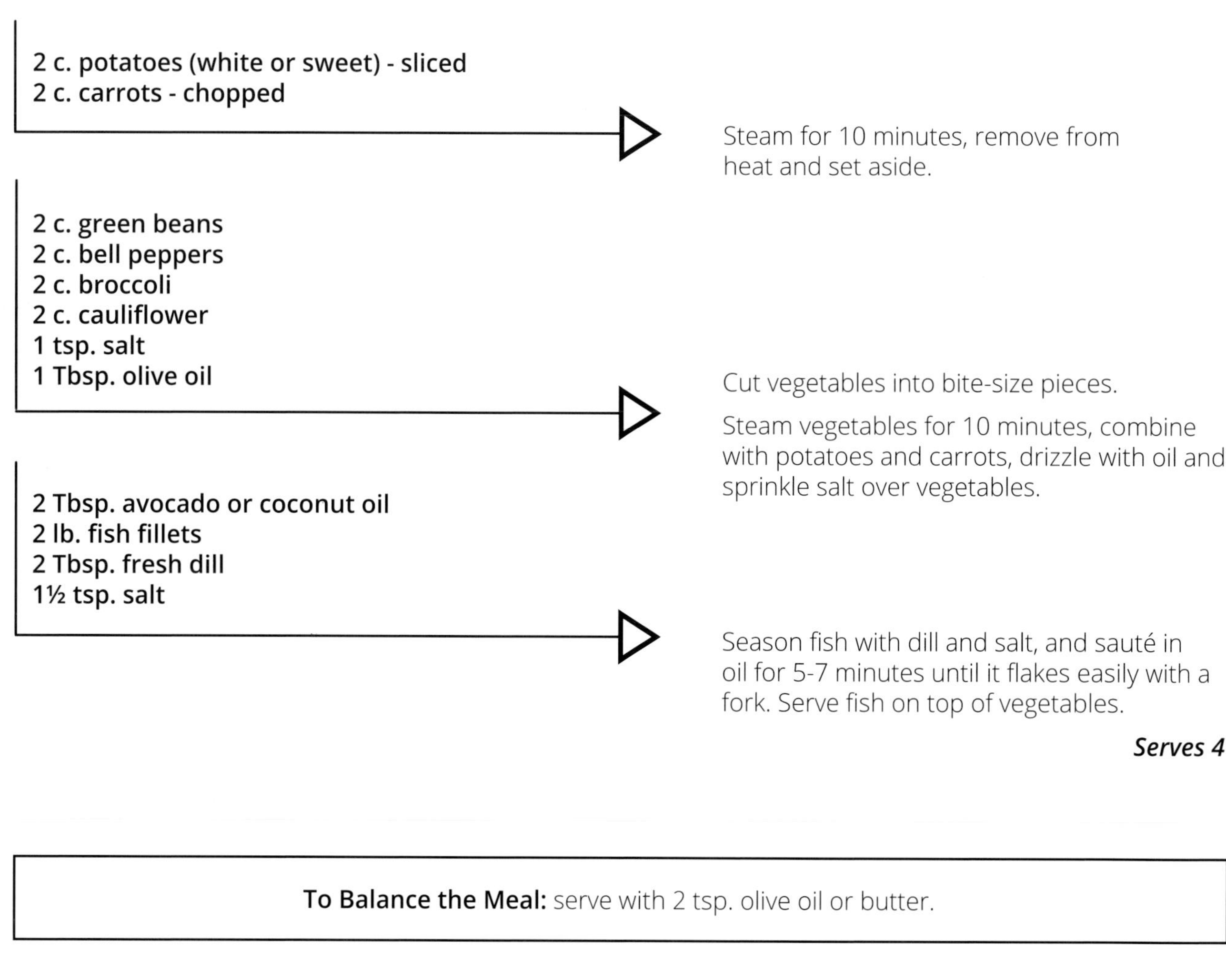

2 c. potatoes (white or sweet) - sliced
2 c. carrots - chopped

Steam for 10 minutes, remove from heat and set aside.

2 c. green beans
2 c. bell peppers
2 c. broccoli
2 c. cauliflower
1 tsp. salt
1 Tbsp. olive oil

Cut vegetables into bite-size pieces.

Steam vegetables for 10 minutes, combine with potatoes and carrots, drizzle with oil and sprinkle salt over vegetables.

2 Tbsp. avocado or coconut oil
2 lb. fish fillets
2 Tbsp. fresh dill
1½ tsp. salt

Season fish with dill and salt, and sauté in oil for 5-7 minutes until it flakes easily with a fork. Serve fish on top of vegetables.

Serves 4

To Balance the Meal: serve with 2 tsp. olive oil or butter.

To make gluten free:
This meal is gluten free

To make dairy free:
Use olive oil instead of butter

Fish Croquettes

6 oz. canned tuna, wild salmon,
 or trout - packed in water, drained
1 egg
4 Wasa Lite Rye crackers - crushed
¼ c. onion - finely chopped
¼ c. celery - finely chopped
Dash onion and/or garlic powder
⅛ tsp. powdered mustard - optional

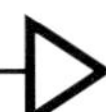

Preheat oven to 350º.

Mix ingredients gently with a fork.

Shape into 8 small cylinders and bake up to 5 minutes on each side until evenly browned.

Serves 2

To Balance the Meal: serve with 1 c. Zucchini Sauté (p. 156).

To make gluten free:
Substitute rice crackers or ½ c. almond meal for Wasa crackers

To make dairy free:
This meal is dairy free

Fish with Lemon and Asparagus

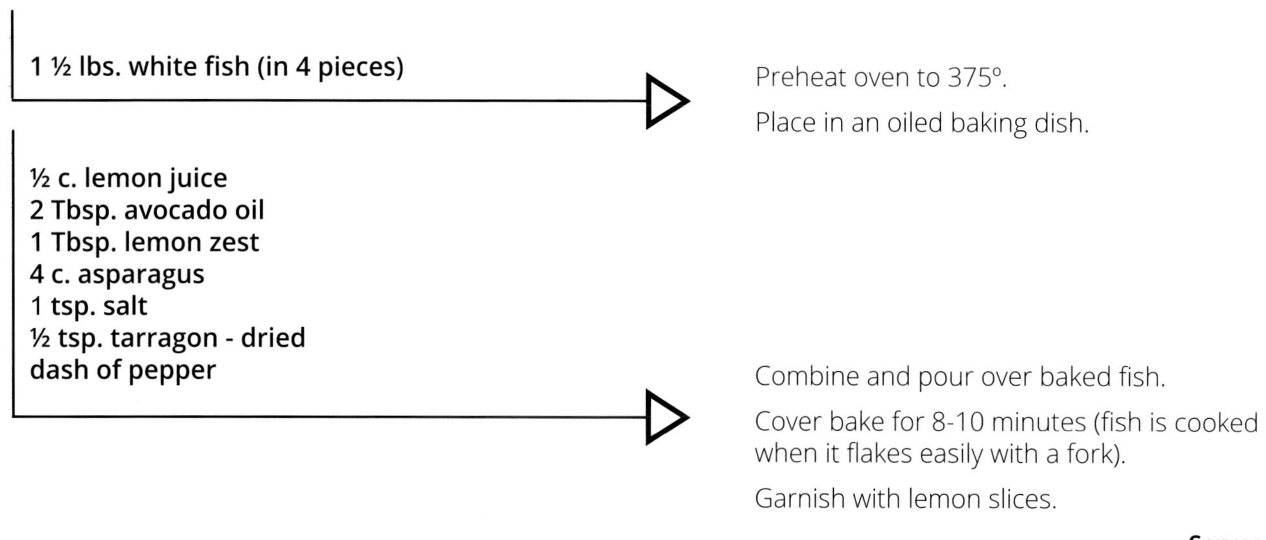

1 ½ lbs. white fish (in 4 pieces)

Preheat oven to 375°.

Place in an oiled baking dish.

½ c. lemon juice
2 Tbsp. avocado oil
1 Tbsp. lemon zest
4 c. asparagus
1 tsp. salt
½ tsp. tarragon - dried
dash of pepper

Combine and pour over baked fish.

Cover bake for 8-10 minutes (fish is cooked when it flakes easily with a fork).

Garnish with lemon slices.

Serves 4

To Balance the Meal: serve with ½ c. wild rice, 2 c. mixed greens and 2 Tbsp. Simple Salad Dressing (p. 134).

To make gluten free:
This meal is gluten free

To make dairy free:
This meal is dairy free

Fresh Shrimp Kabobs

¼ c. white wine vinegar
2 Tbsp. lime juice
2 Tbsp. green onions - sliced
2 Tbsp. avocado oil
1 Tbsp. Dijon mustard
¼ tsp. pepper
½ tsp. salt

Combine these ingredients to make marinade. Set aside ½ of the marinade to be used for basting later.

1¼ lb. large raw shrimp - peeled and deveined

Remove tails from shrimp and place in marinade. Cover and refrigerate for 1 hour.

1 spaghetti squash (3 lb.)

Cut in half lengthwise, discarding seeds. Place cut side down in a Dutch oven. Add 2" of water. Simmer for 20 minutes or until tender. Drain. Remove squash with a spoon or fork.

2 Tbsp. fresh parsley - chopped
2 Tbsp. butter
½ tsp. salt

Spread squash on serving plate and top with parsley and butter, and season with salt.

Keep warm.

8 large mushroom caps
1 zucchini - sliced ½" thick
2 sweet red peppers - cut into 1" pieces
½ onion - cut in 1" pieces

Preheat grill to medium high. Remove shrimp from marinade.

Place shrimp and veggies on separate skewers.

Grill uncovered 4 minutes on each side, basting with the marinade that was set aside, until shrimp is done.

Serve skewers over squash.

Serves 4

To Balance the Meal: this meal is balanced.

To make gluten free:
This meal is gluten free

To make dairy free:
Use coconut oil instead of butter

Salmon Loaf

3, 7.5-oz. cans salmon
1 c. wild rice or steel cut oats - cooked
1 tsp. salt
1 tsp. black pepper
½ c. cream
2 eggs

Preheat oven to 350°.

Mix well and let stand.

½ c. green pepper - diced
½ c. onion - diced
1 tsp. avocado or coconut oil

Heat a small sauté, add oil and cook until tender. Let cool slightly.

Mix vegetables with salmon mixture.

Place mixture in an oiled 8" loaf pan.

Bake 40 minutes until golden brown

Serves 4

To Balance the Meal: serve with a large green salad with 1 Tbsp. Simple Salad Dressing (p. 134) or 2 c. vegetables with 2 tsp. butter.

To make gluten free:
This meal is gluten free

To make dairy free:
Use canned coconut milk instead of cream

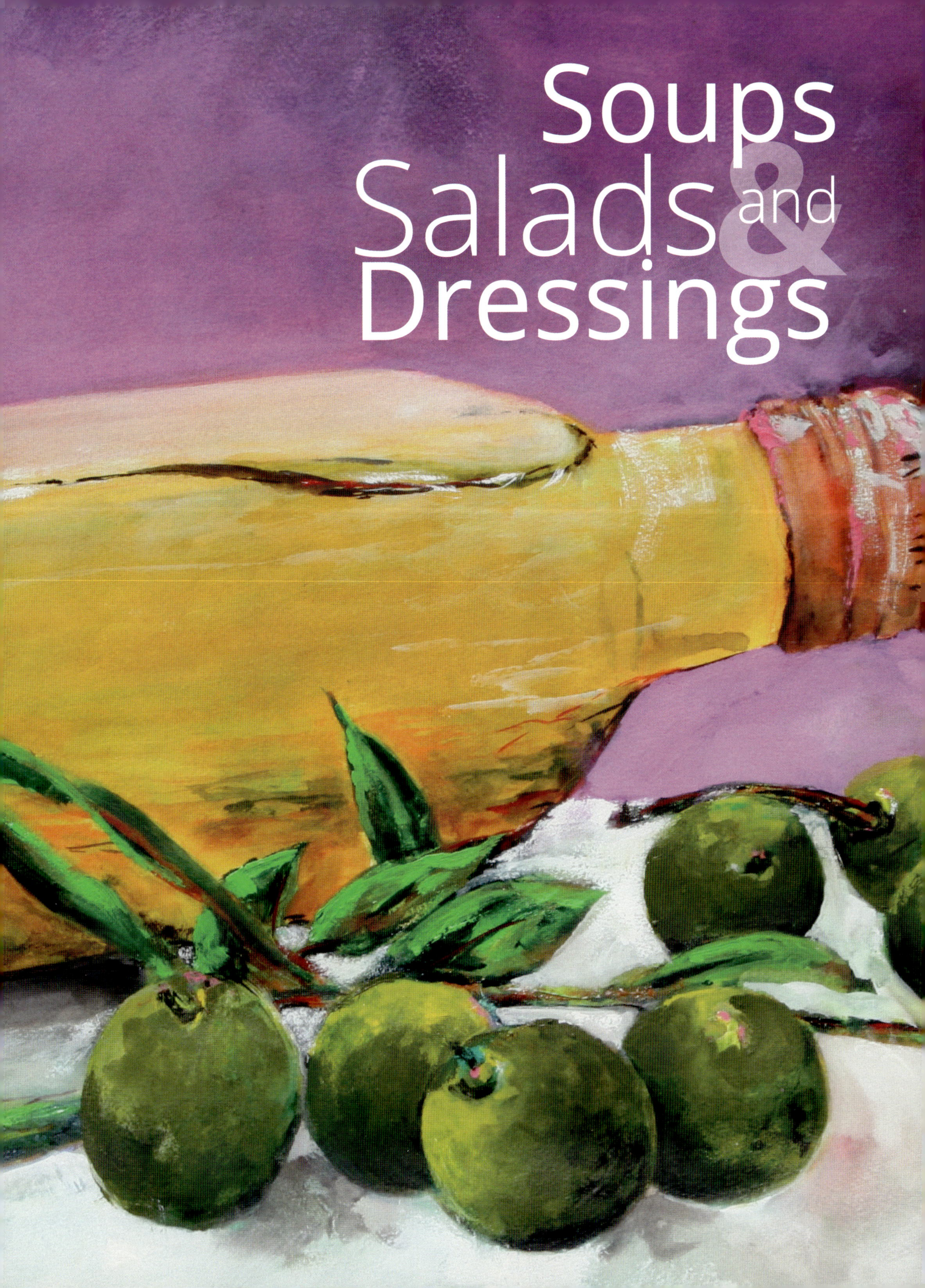
Soups
Salads and
& Dressings

Bone-Building Broth

1 lb. bones from a free range animal
(chicken, beef, ham bone, etc.)
4 qt. water
2 Tbsp. vinegar
2 large onions - cut in half
3 carrots - cut into large pieces
4 celery stalks - cut into large pieces
8 whole cloves garlic
3 parsnips - cut into large pieces
10 fresh sprigs of thyme
10 whole peppercorns

Place bones, water and vinegar in a large pot. Let sit for 30-60 minutes.

Add remaining ingredients and bring to a boil. Cover, reduce heat and simmer for at least 4 hours or up to 12 hours. Periodically scoop off foam that rises to the top and discard.

Strain stock into a large bowl, keep refrigerated or freeze for later use.

The same steps can be used with a crockpot set on low for 8-12 hours.

Tip: freeze broth in an ice cube tray or muffin tin for later use in small amounts.

To Balance the Meal: use broth in Bone-Building Chicken Soup (p. 104).

To make gluten free:
This is gluten free

To make dairy free:
This is dairy free

Bone-Building Chicken Soup

1 Tbsp. olive oil
2 leeks - cleaned and thinly sliced
6 cloves garlic - minced
2 qt. chicken stock
2 c. celery - chopped
2 carrots - peeled and chopped
3 parsnips - peeled and chopped
1 c. frozen peas
1 c. frozen green beans
1 tsp. dried thyme
2 tsp. sea salt
½ tsp. ground black pepper

In a stock pot, heat oil on medium heat and sauté leeks and garlic for 2 minutes. Add stock, remaining vegetables and seasonings. Bring to a simmer for 20-30 minutes until vegetables are tender.

1 lb. cooked chicken - shredded or cubed
2 c. spinach or kale - chopped

Stir chicken and spinach or kale into soup and simmer for 10 minutes.

Serves 4-6

To Balance the Meal: top each bowl of soup with freshly minced parsley and 6 chopped olives.

To make gluten free:
This is gluten free

To make dairy free:
This is dairy free

Chicken Vegetable Soup

2 Tbsp. avocado or coconut oil
1 c. onion - diced
1 clove garlic - minced
4 c. cooked chicken - diced

In a 4-quart sauce pan, sauté onion and garlic in oil and add cooked chicken.

4 c. chicken broth - preservative free
½ c. quinoa - uncooked
2 c. fresh tomato - diced
1 tsp. salt
½ tsp. dried thyme
1 tsp. dried basil leaves
¼ tsp. red pepper flakes

Add broth and stir in remaining ingredients.

Bring to a boil, reduce heat and simmer for 30 minutes or until quinoa is tender.

1½ c. mixed vegetables - fresh or frozen

Add and heat until warm.

Serves 4

To Balance the Meal: serve with celery and carrot sticks and 1-2 Tbsp. real nut butter.

To make gluten free:
This meal is gluten free

To make dairy free:
This meal is dairy free

Chicken Wild Rice Soup

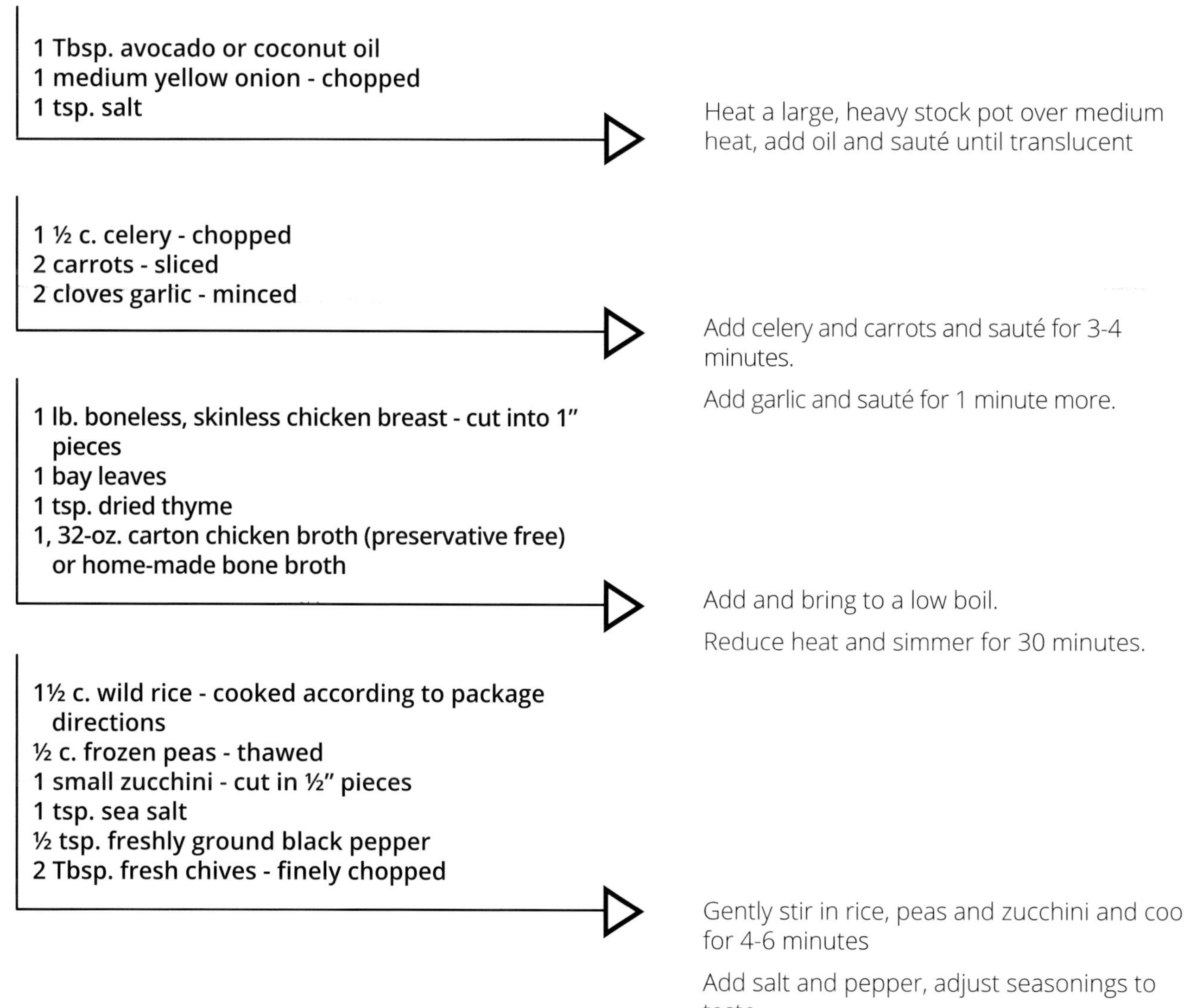

1 Tbsp. avocado or coconut oil
1 medium yellow onion - chopped
1 tsp. salt

Heat a large, heavy stock pot over medium heat, add oil and sauté until translucent

1 ½ c. celery - chopped
2 carrots - sliced
2 cloves garlic - minced

Add celery and carrots and sauté for 3-4 minutes.

Add garlic and sauté for 1 minute more.

1 lb. boneless, skinless chicken breast - cut into 1" pieces
1 bay leaves
1 tsp. dried thyme
1, 32-oz. carton chicken broth (preservative free) or home-made bone broth

Add and bring to a low boil.

Reduce heat and simmer for 30 minutes.

1½ c. wild rice - cooked according to package directions
½ c. frozen peas - thawed
1 small zucchini - cut in ½" pieces
1 tsp. sea salt
½ tsp. freshly ground black pepper
2 Tbsp. fresh chives - finely chopped

Gently stir in rice, peas and zucchini and cook for 4-6 minutes

Add salt and pepper, adjust seasonings to taste.

Garnish with chives.

Serves 4

To Balance the Meal: serve with celery and 1-2 Tbsp. cream cheese or 2 Wasa crackers and 1 Tbsp. cream cheese.

To make gluten free:
This meal is gluten free

To make dairy free:
Replace cream cheese with nut butter

Salmon Chowder

1 Tbsp. avocado oil or ghee
1 medium onion - chopped
½ c. celery - chopped

Melt oil or ghee in a large soup pot. Add onion and celery. Sauté 5 minutes.

1 Tbsp. corn starch
3 c. chicken broth, divided

Stir corn starch into ¼ c. of the chicken broth and set aside.

2 small red potatoes
½ tsp. salt
¼ tsp. ground black pepper
1 lb. salmon fillets - skin removed, cut into bite-size pieces
12 oz. green beans - cut into bite-size pieces
½ c. frozen corn
1-2 c. whole milk or half & half

Pour remaining broth into pot and simmer. Add potatoes, salt, and pepper and simmer for 15 minutes. Add salmon and remaining vegetables to the pot. Simmer for 10 minutes. Stir in cornstarch mixture and simmer another 3-5 minutes as soup thickens and green beans finish cooking.

Stir in milk. Heat until warm.

Serve with chopped fresh parsley or dill.

Serves 4

To Balance the Meal: this meal is balanced.

To make gluten free:
This is gluten free

To make dairy free:
Subsitute coconut milk for whole milk or half and half

Sausage, White Bean and Kale Minestrone

3 Tbsp. avocado or coconut oil
2 c. onion - coarsely chopped
2 red bell pepper - coarsely chopped

Cook in a large soup pot over medium heat, stirring occasionally, until onion is translucent, about 8 minutes.

2 cloves garlic - minced

Add and cook 1 minute.

8 c. chicken broth
2 medium carrots - chopped
1 c. celery - chopped
1 bay leaf
1 tsp. thyme - dried
1 tsp. basil - dried

Add to pot.

Bring to boil, then reduce heat to medium low and simmer about 10-15 minutes.

16-oz. bag chopped kale
1, 15-oz. can white beans - drained, rinsed
2 lbs. nitrate-free turkey or chicken sausage - sliced
1, 28-oz. can diced tomatoes
24 olives - chopped (black or kalamata)
2 Tbsp. tomato paste
2½ tsp. salt
½ - 1½ tsp. ground black pepper
½ c. packed fresh parsley - chopped

Add remaining ingredients, except parsley, salt and pepper, and simmer for 25 minutes.

Add seasonings to taste, remove bay leaf and stir in parsley just before serving.

Serves 6

To Balance the Meal: this meal is balanced.

To make gluten free:
This meal is gluten free

To make dairy free:
This meal is dairy free

Build a Balanced *Salad*

STEP 1: *Choose a healthy protein (4-6 oz.)*

Beef patty	Turkey	Steak	Salmon
Chicken breast	Shrimp	Tuna	Eggs

STEP 2: *Choose a variety of healthy carbs*

Unlimited vegetables (1-3 c.):

Fresh salad greens	Cucumbers
Peppers	Cauliflower
Green beans	Mushrooms
Tomatoes	Zucchini
Broccoli	Snap peas

Limited carbs (½ c.):

Beans	Sweet potatoes
Peas	Raspberries
Corn	Strawberries
Carrots	Pears
Wild rice	Apples

STEP 3: *Choose a healthy fat*

Olive oil (1 T.)

Nuts (¼ c.)

Seeds (2 T.)

Avocado (½)

Cold-pressed mayonnaise (1-2 T.)

Olives (6-10)

OPTIONAL: Add additional flavor (1-2 T.)

Cheese such as feta, blue cheese, parmesan, mozzarella or cheddar

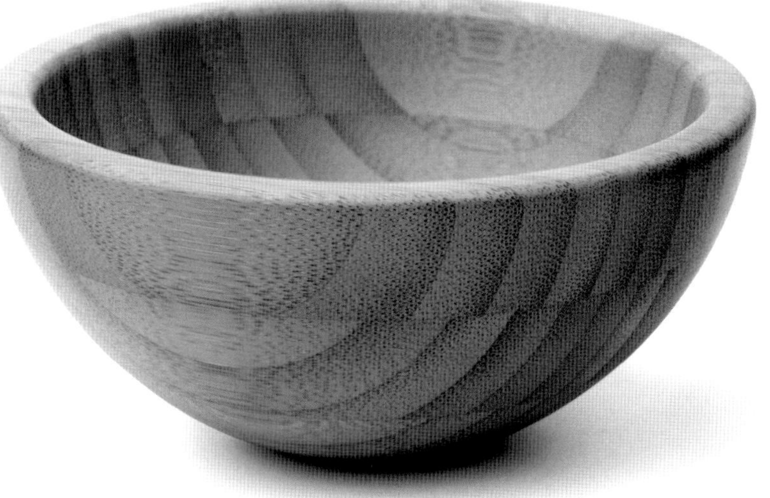

Almond-Crusted Chicken Salad

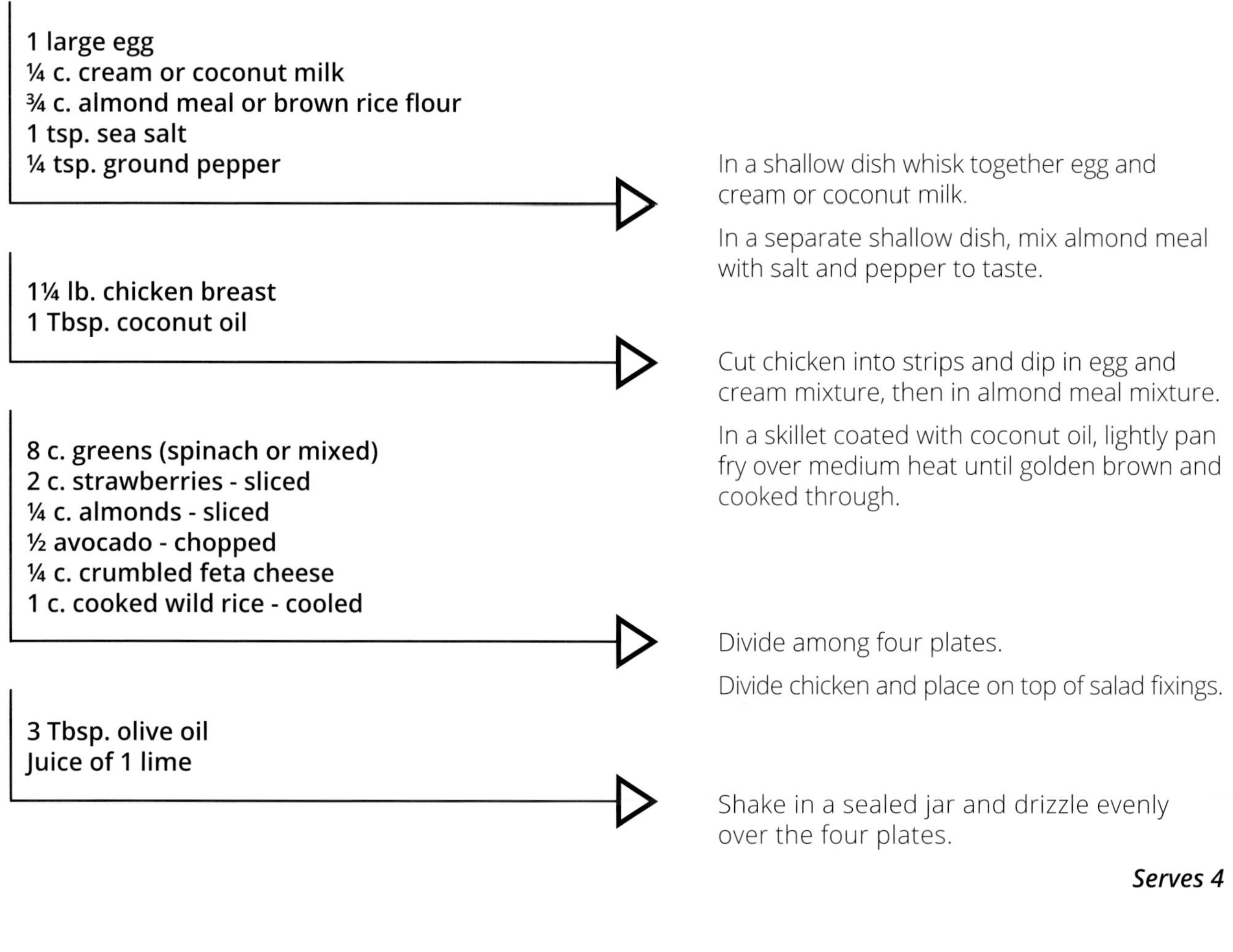

1 large egg
¼ c. cream or coconut milk
¾ c. almond meal or brown rice flour
1 tsp. sea salt
¼ tsp. ground pepper

In a shallow dish whisk together egg and cream or coconut milk.

In a separate shallow dish, mix almond meal with salt and pepper to taste.

1¼ lb. chicken breast
1 Tbsp. coconut oil

Cut chicken into strips and dip in egg and cream mixture, then in almond meal mixture.

In a skillet coated with coconut oil, lightly pan fry over medium heat until golden brown and cooked through.

8 c. greens (spinach or mixed)
2 c. strawberries - sliced
¼ c. almonds - sliced
½ avocado - chopped
¼ c. crumbled feta cheese
1 c. cooked wild rice - cooled

Divide among four plates.

Divide chicken and place on top of salad fixings.

3 Tbsp. olive oil
Juice of 1 lime

Shake in a sealed jar and drizzle evenly over the four plates.

Serves 4

To Balance the Meal: this meal is balanced.

To make gluten free:
This meal is gluten free

To make dairy free:
Use coconut milk instead of cream and omit feta cheese

Artichoke-Caper-Lemon Tuna Salad

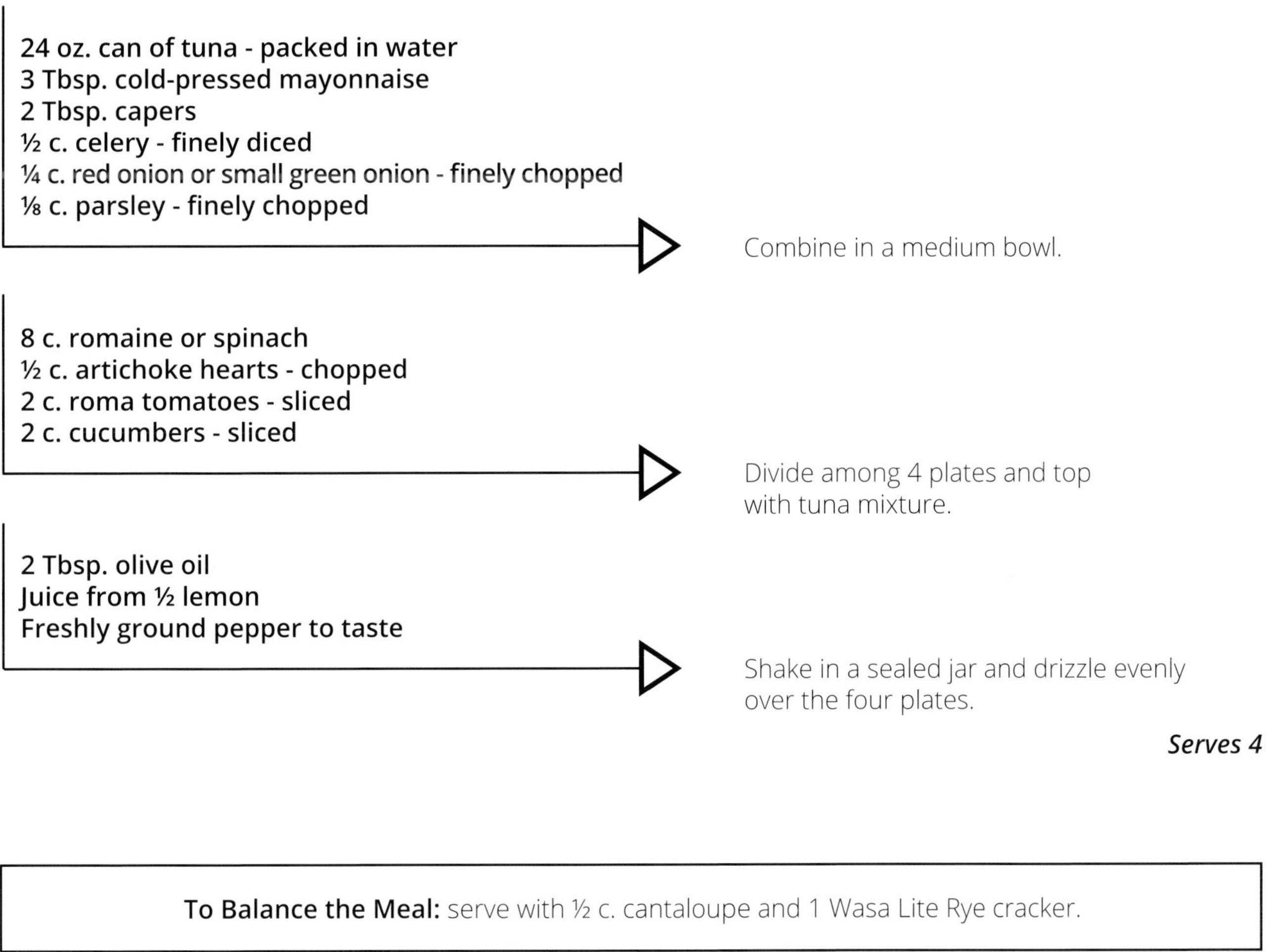

24 oz. can of tuna - packed in water
3 Tbsp. cold-pressed mayonnaise
2 Tbsp. capers
½ c. celery - finely diced
¼ c. red onion or small green onion - finely chopped
⅛ c. parsley - finely chopped

Combine in a medium bowl.

8 c. romaine or spinach
½ c. artichoke hearts - chopped
2 c. roma tomatoes - sliced
2 c. cucumbers - sliced

Divide among 4 plates and top with tuna mixture.

2 Tbsp. olive oil
Juice from ½ lemon
Freshly ground pepper to taste

Shake in a sealed jar and drizzle evenly over the four plates.

Serves 4

To Balance the Meal: serve with ½ c. cantaloupe and 1 Wasa Lite Rye cracker.

To make gluten free:
Use gluten-free crackers

To make dairy free:
This meal is dairy free

Asian Salmon Salad

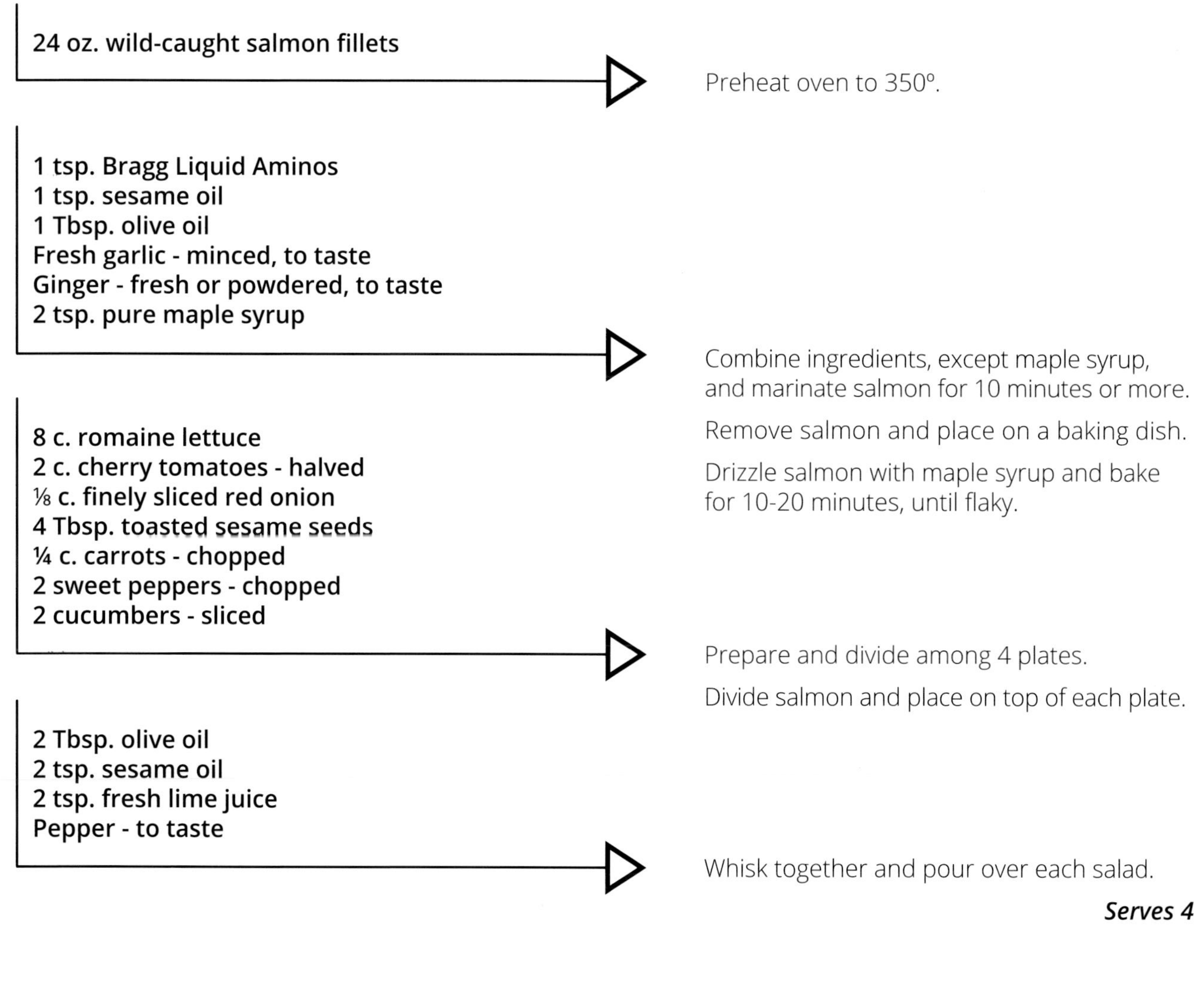

To Balance the Meal: serve with 1 kiwi fruit.

To make gluten free:
This meal is gluten free

To make dairy free:
This meal is dairy free

Avocado-Tomato Chutney

2 avocados - scooped out of the skin
and chopped
6 roma tomatoes - chopped
¼ c. red onion - chopped
½ c. pineapple - chopped
2 Tbsp. olive oil
Dash lime juice
2 Tbsp. fresh cilantro or basil - chopped
Sea salt and pepper to taste

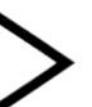

Combine all ingredients and serve.

Serves 4

To Balance the Meal: serve over the top of a grilled Bison Burger (p. 50) and ½ c. pineapple.

To make gluten free:
This meal is gluten free

To make dairy free:
This meal is dairy free

Chicken Salad with Apples

½ c. cold-pressed mayonnaise
1 Tbsp. lemon juice
Dash of salt
Dash of onion salt
16 oz. chicken breast - cooked and cubed
1½ c. apples - diced
1½ c. celery - diced

Whisk mayonnaise, lemon juice and seasonings together.

Mix in remaining ingredients and serve.

Serves 4

To Balance the Meal: serve on a bed of greens.

To make gluten free:
This meal is gluten free

To make dairy free:
This meal is dairy free

Chickpea Salad with Sardines

½ c. canned chickpeas (garbanzo beans) - drained and rinsed
1 small cucumber - chopped
2 small tomatoes - chopped
1 Tbsp. olive oil
Juice of ½ lemon
1, 4-oz. can of sardines - in water or olive oil, drained (or 4 oz. tuna)
Salt and pepper to taste
¼ c. chopped fresh parsley

Combine all ingredients in a bowl. Eat immediately or allow to marinate overnight.

Serves 1

To Balance the Meal: This meal is balanced.

To make gluten free:
This is gluten free

To make dairy free:
This is dairy free

Crunchy Broccoli Salad

½ c. cold-pressed mayonnaise
1 Tbsp. apple cider vinegar
¼ tsp. black pepper
1 tsp. salt

→ Mix in a large bowl.

6 c. broccoli - cut into bite-size pieces

→ Add to mayonnaise dressing and toss.

4 slices bacon - cooked and diced
2 c. red grapes - sliced in half
¼ c. slivered almonds
¼ c. red onion - diced (optional)

→ Add to broccoli mixture & toss together.

Serves 4

To Balance the Meal: serve with 4 oz. beef roast.

To make gluten free:
This is gluten free

To make dairy free:
This is dairy free

Fact *VS.* **Fiction**

Fiction	Fact
Bread has fiber, and I need fiber.	Most bread has 2-3 grams of fiber per slice. Compare that to a cup of broccoli that has 5 grams. Broccoli and other vegetables are the best sources of fiber.

Cucumber Salad with Curried Chicken

1 Tbsp. coconut oil (or ghee)
1 ½ tsp. curry powder (or garam masala)
¼ tsp. salt
Pepper to taste
8 oz. chicken tenders

Heat oil in a skillet over medium-high heat.

Add curry and stir briefly.

Season chicken with salt and pepper and add to the pan, coating with the curry oil. Saute until cooked through about 4 – 6 minutes. Remove and set aside.

1 tsp. coconut oil (or ghee)
½ small onion - diced
2 bell peppers (red or green) - chopped
1 tsp. ginger - grated
1 c. brown rice - cooked
¼ tsp. salt

In the same pan, heat the oil and add the onion and peppers and sauté until translucent. Add the ginger and the rice and stir well to combine. Cook until heated through and season with salt.

2 Tbsp. avocado oil
1 Tbsp. rice vinegar
1 tsp. coconut aminos
6 c. romaine lettuce - chopped
¼ c. chopped fresh herbs - mint, basil, parsley
2 c. cucumber - sliced
½ avocado - sliced

In a large bowl, whisk the oil, vinegar and coconut aminos until well combined.

Add the chopped romaine and herbs and toss to coat with the dressing.

Divide the salad greens between two shallow bowls and top with the chicken, rice mixture and fan out the cucumbers and avocado slices.

Serves 2

To Balance the Meal: this meal is balanced.

To make gluten free:
This meal is gluten free

To make dairy free:
This meal is dairy free

Easy Chopped Salad

8 c. field greens
4 oz. mozzarella - diced or shredded
1 c. artichoke hearts - sliced
1½ c. carrots - chopped
2 c. celery - chopped
2 c. cherry tomatoes - halved
18 oz. shrimp or chicken - cooked and cut into bite-sized pieces
1 c. corn - fresh or frozen

Combine in a large bowl.

1 tsp. dijon
¼ c. olive oil
3 Tbsp. balsamic vinegar
Sea salt and pepper to taste

Whisk together, then toss with salad and serve.

Serves 4

To Balance the Meal: this meal is balanced.

To make gluten free:
This meal is gluten free

To make dairy free:
Omit mozzarella and add 4 oz. additional shrimp or chicken

Easy Salmon Salad

½ tsp. salt
1, 7.5-oz. can water-packed salmon - drained
½ c. celery - diced
2 Tbsp. green onion - chopped
½ c. peas - fresh or frozen
1 hard boiled egg - chopped
5 large ripe olives - sliced
3 Tbsp. cold-pressed mayonnaise
2 Tbsp. fresh tarragon
Squeeze of fresh lemon

Combine in a large bowl.

Serves 2

To Balance the Meal: serve over 2 c. salad greens with 1-2 Wasa lite rye crackers.

To make gluten free:
Use gluten-free crackers

To make dairy free:
This meal is dairy free

Jicama Salad

1 medium jicama - peeled and thinly sliced
1 red pepper - thinly sliced
1 green pepper - thinly sliced
1 yellow pepper - thinly sliced
1 cucumber - diced
¼ c. lime juice
1/3 c. olive oil
½ c. fresh cilantro - chopped (optional)
Salt and pepper to taste

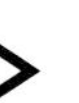

Combine all ingredients in a large bowl and let marinate 1-4 hours.

Serves 6-8

To Balance the Meal: serve with 4 oz. Instant Pot Citrus Pork (p. 76) and ½ sweet potato with 1 tsp. butter.

To make gluten free:
This is gluten free

To make dairy free:
Replace butter with coconut oil

Mediterranean Potato Salad

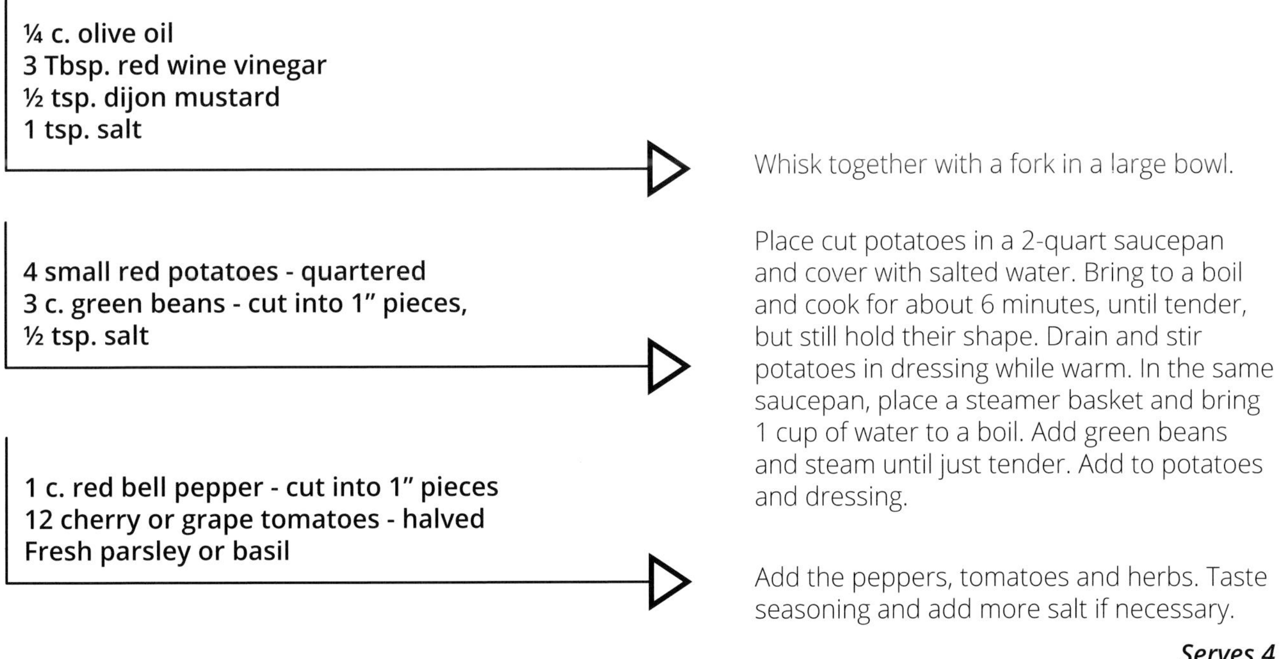

¼ c. olive oil
3 Tbsp. red wine vinegar
½ tsp. dijon mustard
1 tsp. salt

Whisk together with a fork in a large bowl.

4 small red potatoes - quartered
3 c. green beans - cut into 1" pieces,
½ tsp. salt

Place cut potatoes in a 2-quart saucepan and cover with salted water. Bring to a boil and cook for about 6 minutes, until tender, but still hold their shape. Drain and stir potatoes in dressing while warm. In the same saucepan, place a steamer basket and bring 1 cup of water to a boil. Add green beans and steam until just tender. Add to potatoes and dressing.

1 c. red bell pepper - cut into 1" pieces
12 cherry or grape tomatoes - halved
Fresh parsley or basil

Add the peppers, tomatoes and herbs. Taste seasoning and add more salt if necessary.

Serves 4

To Balance the Meal: serve with 4 oz. steak.

To make gluten free:
This is gluten free

To make dairy free:
This is dairy free

Quinoa Salad with Turkey

½ c. quinoa - uncooked
1 c. water or broth

Rinse quinoa well, then drain.

Combine with water in a 2-quart saucepan, bring to a boil, then simmer covered for 5 minutes. Remove from heat and keep covered for 15-20 minutes, or until all of the water is absorbed. Allow to cool.

¾ lb. cooked turkey breast
1 c. celery - chopped
1 c. red pepper - chopped
¼ c. green onion - sliced
3 Tbsp. olive oil
¼ c. lime juice
Fresh cilantro - chopped (to taste)
½ tsp. chili powder

In a large bowl, combine these ingredients with cooled quinoa.

Refrigerate for 1-2 hours to allow flavors to blend.

When ready to serve, spoon onto a romaine leaf for garnish.

Serves 3

To Balance the Meal: this meal is balanced.

To make gluten free:
This meal is gluten free

To make dairy free:
This meal is dairy free

Sonoma Chicken Salad

2 c. rotisserie chicken - diced
1 c. celery - diced
2 Tbsp. cold-pressed mayonnaise
1 tsp. apple cider vinegar
2 tsp. pure maple syrup (optional)

Mix in a large bowl.

20 grapes - sliced in half
¼ c. pecans - chopped
1 tsp. poppy seeds

Add and stir.

Serves 2

To Balance the Meal: serve over mixed greens or baby spinach with sliced cucumbers and tomatoes.

To make gluten free:
This is gluten free

To make dairy free:
This is dairy free

Southwestern Chili Salad

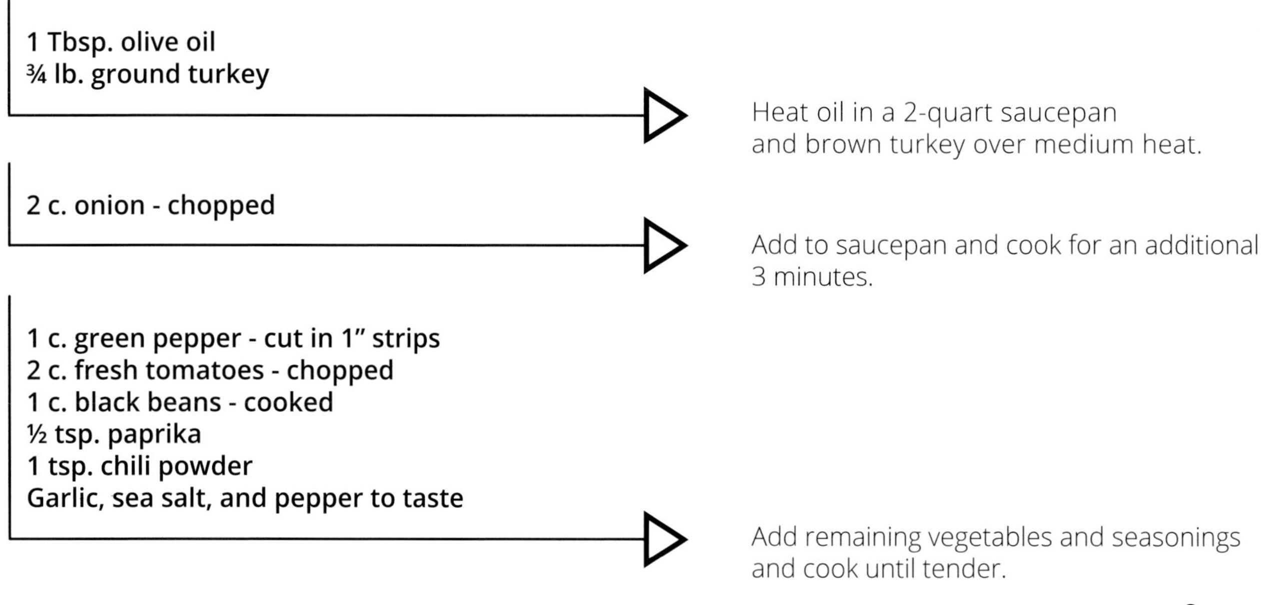

1 Tbsp. olive oil
¾ lb. ground turkey
Heat oil in a 2-quart saucepan and brown turkey over medium heat.
2 c. onion - chopped
Add to saucepan and cook for an additional 3 minutes.
1 c. green pepper - cut in 1" strips
2 c. fresh tomatoes - chopped
1 c. black beans - cooked
½ tsp. paprika
1 tsp. chili powder
Garlic, sea salt, and pepper to taste
Add remaining vegetables and seasonings and cook until tender.

Serves 2

To Balance the Meal: serve over 2 c. romaine leaves and 1 c. vegetables. Top with 1 Tbsp. sour cream or ½ avocado.

To make gluten free:
This meal is gluten free

To make dairy free:
Use ½ avocado instead of sour cream

Spinach Salad with Chicken

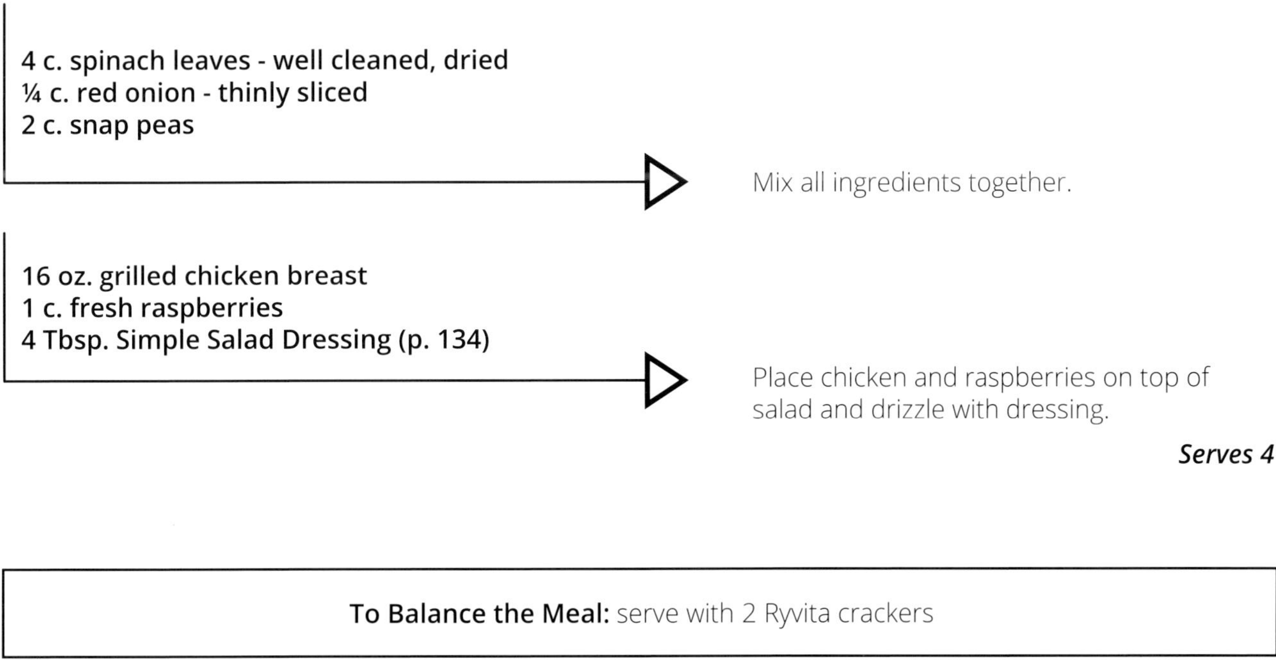

4 c. spinach leaves - well cleaned, dried
¼ c. red onion - thinly sliced
2 c. snap peas

Mix all ingredients together.

16 oz. grilled chicken breast
1 c. fresh raspberries
4 Tbsp. Simple Salad Dressing (p. 134)

Place chicken and raspberries on top of salad and drizzle with dressing.

Serves 4

To Balance the Meal: serve with 2 Ryvita crackers

To make gluten free:
Use gluten-free crackers

To make dairy free:
This meal is dairy free

Steak Salad with Gorgonzola

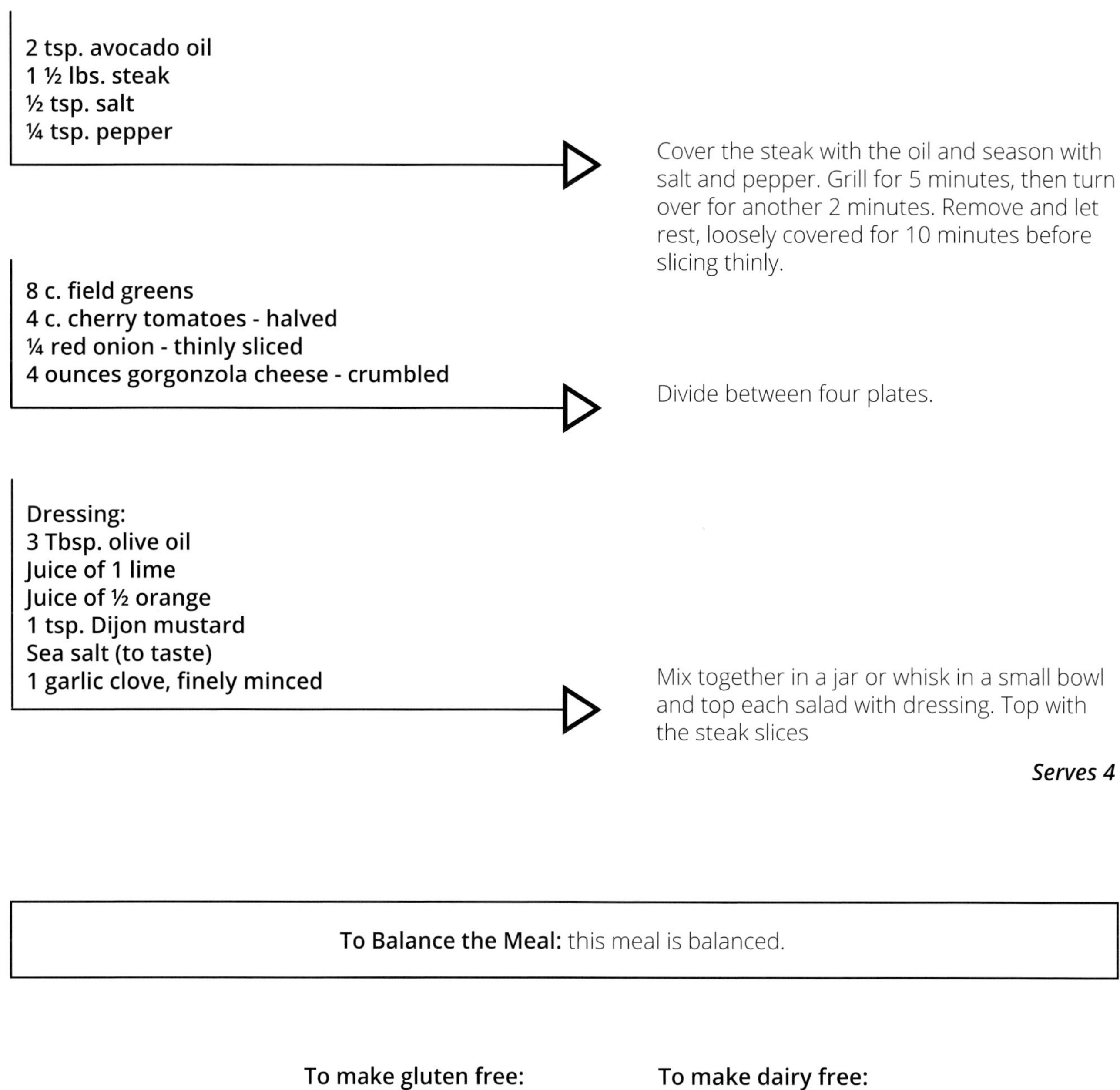

2 tsp. avocado oil
1 ½ lbs. steak
½ tsp. salt
¼ tsp. pepper

Cover the steak with the oil and season with salt and pepper. Grill for 5 minutes, then turn over for another 2 minutes. Remove and let rest, loosely covered for 10 minutes before slicing thinly.

8 c. field greens
4 c. cherry tomatoes - halved
¼ red onion - thinly sliced
4 ounces gorgonzola cheese - crumbled

Divide between four plates.

Dressing:
3 Tbsp. olive oil
Juice of 1 lime
Juice of ½ orange
1 tsp. Dijon mustard
Sea salt (to taste)
1 garlic clove, finely minced

Mix together in a jar or whisk in a small bowl and top each salad with dressing. Top with the steak slices

Serves 4

To Balance the Meal: this meal is balanced.

To make gluten free:
This meal is gluten free

To make dairy free:
Omit gorgonzola cheese

Tex-Mex Turkey Salad

1 Tbsp. olive oil
¼ tsp. salt
½ tsp. paprika
¼ tsp. chili powder
¼ tsp. cumin
Juice of 1 lime
½ c. salsa
½ c. corn - fresh or frozen

Combine in a bowl.

8 oz. cooked turkey breast - cut into ½" cubes

Add turkey to the bowl and mix thoroughly.

1 head romaine lettuce
2 Tbsp. salsa

Divide lettuce into two portions and arrange on dinner plates.

Spoon half of turkey mixture over each plate of greens and top with salsa.

Serves 2

To Balance the Meal: this meal is balanced.

To make gluten free:
This meal is gluten free

To make dairy free:
This meal is dairy free

Tofu Cauliflower Egg Salad

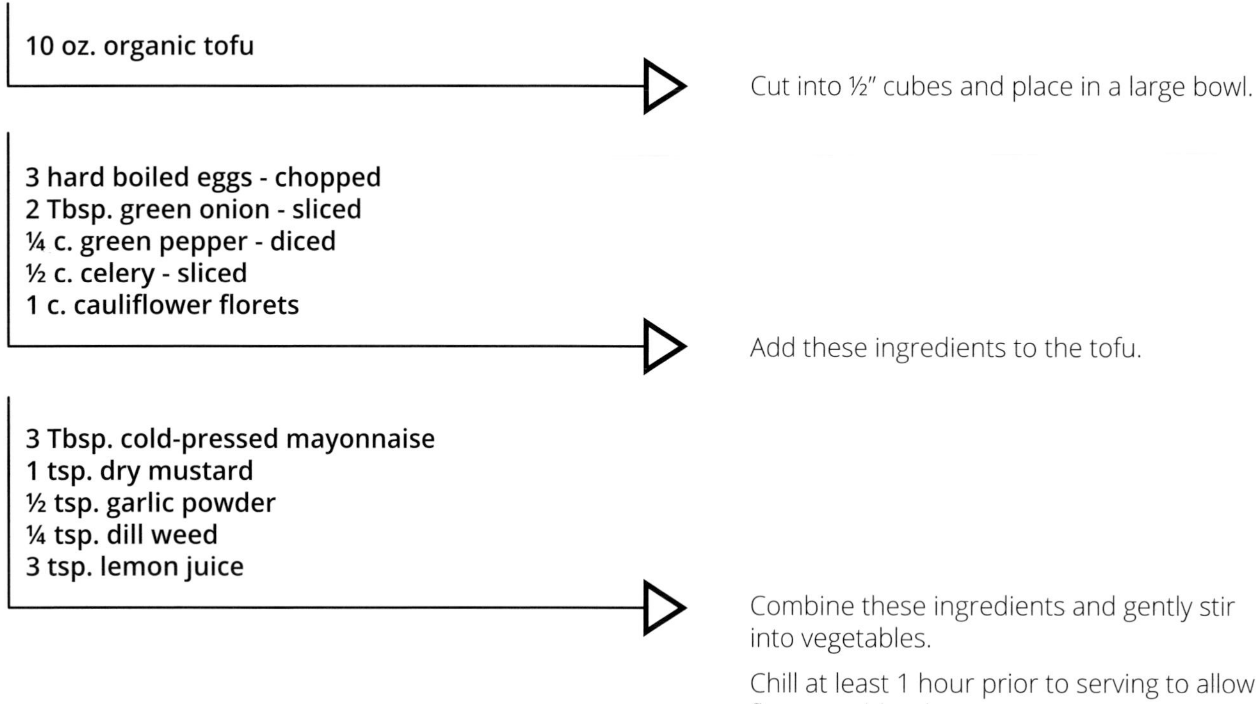
10 oz. organic tofu

Cut into ½" cubes and place in a large bowl.

3 hard boiled eggs - chopped
2 Tbsp. green onion - sliced
¼ c. green pepper - diced
½ c. celery - sliced
1 c. cauliflower florets

Add these ingredients to the tofu.

3 Tbsp. cold-pressed mayonnaise
1 tsp. dry mustard
½ tsp. garlic powder
¼ tsp. dill weed
3 tsp. lemon juice

Combine these ingredients and gently stir into vegetables.

Chill at least 1 hour prior to serving to allow flavors to blend.

Serves 2

To Balance the Meal: serve with 2 Wasa Lite Rye crackers and 1 Tbsp. almond butter.

To make gluten free:
Use gluten-free crackers

To make dairy free:
This meal is dairy free

Traditional Greek Salad

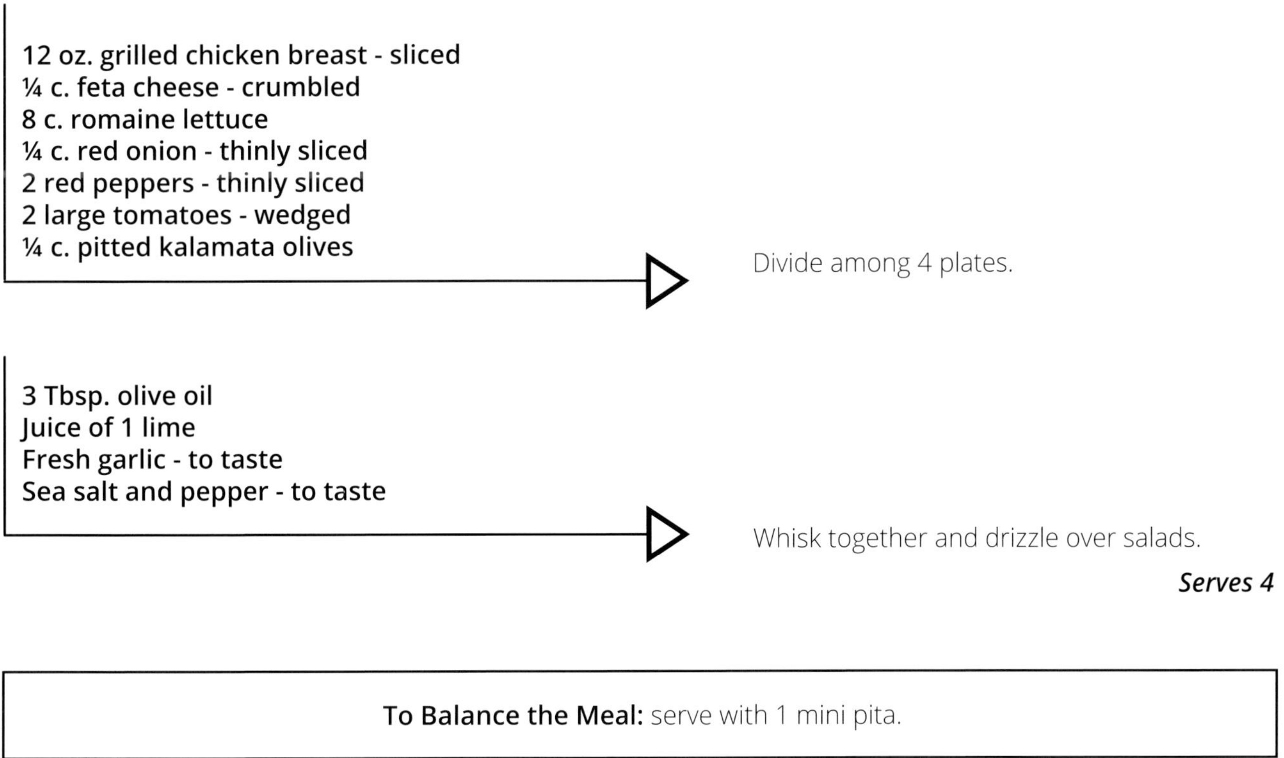

12 oz. grilled chicken breast - sliced
¼ c. feta cheese - crumbled
8 c. romaine lettuce
¼ c. red onion - thinly sliced
2 red peppers - thinly sliced
2 large tomatoes - wedged
¼ c. pitted kalamata olives
Divide among 4 plates.
3 Tbsp. olive oil
Juice of 1 lime
Fresh garlic - to taste
Sea salt and pepper - to taste
Whisk together and drizzle over salads.

Serves 4

To Balance the Meal: serve with 1 mini pita.

To make gluten free:
Serve with a gluten-free pita or tortilla

To make dairy free:
Omit feta cheese

Tuna-Stuffed Tomatoes

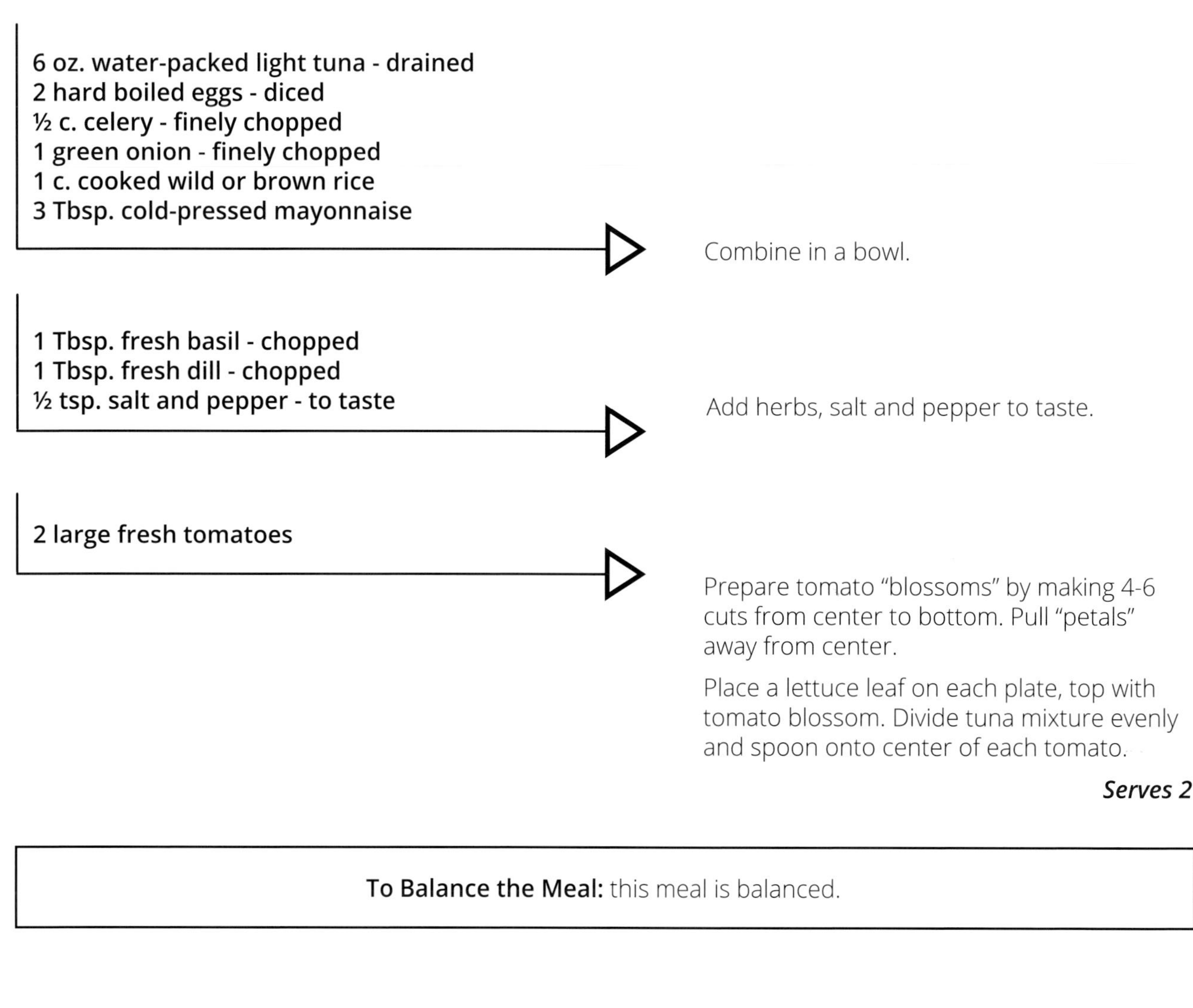

6 oz. water-packed light tuna - drained
2 hard boiled eggs - diced
½ c. celery - finely chopped
1 green onion - finely chopped
1 c. cooked wild or brown rice
3 Tbsp. cold-pressed mayonnaise

Combine in a bowl.

1 Tbsp. fresh basil - chopped
1 Tbsp. fresh dill - chopped
½ tsp. salt and pepper - to taste

Add herbs, salt and pepper to taste.

2 large fresh tomatoes

Prepare tomato "blossoms" by making 4-6 cuts from center to bottom. Pull "petals" away from center.

Place a lettuce leaf on each plate, top with tomato blossom. Divide tuna mixture evenly and spoon onto center of each tomato.

Serves 2

To Balance the Meal: this meal is balanced.

To make gluten free:
This meal is gluten free

To make dairy free:
This meal is dairy free

Turkey Avocado Cobb Salad

8 c. mixed greens
2 c. cherry tomatoes - sliced
1 avocado - sliced
4 slices nitrate-free bacon - cooked, crumbled
10 oz. cooked turkey or chicken - diced
2 hard-boiled eggs - sliced
2 Tbsp. green onions - sliced
2 c. white potato - cooked

Combine in a large bowl.

3 Tbsp. olive oil
Juice of 1 lime
Ground pepper - to taste

Add to ingredients in bowl, divide among plates and serve.

Serves 4

To Balance the Meal: this meal is balanced.

To make gluten free:
This meal is gluten free

To make dairy free:
This meal is dairy free

Fay's Salsa

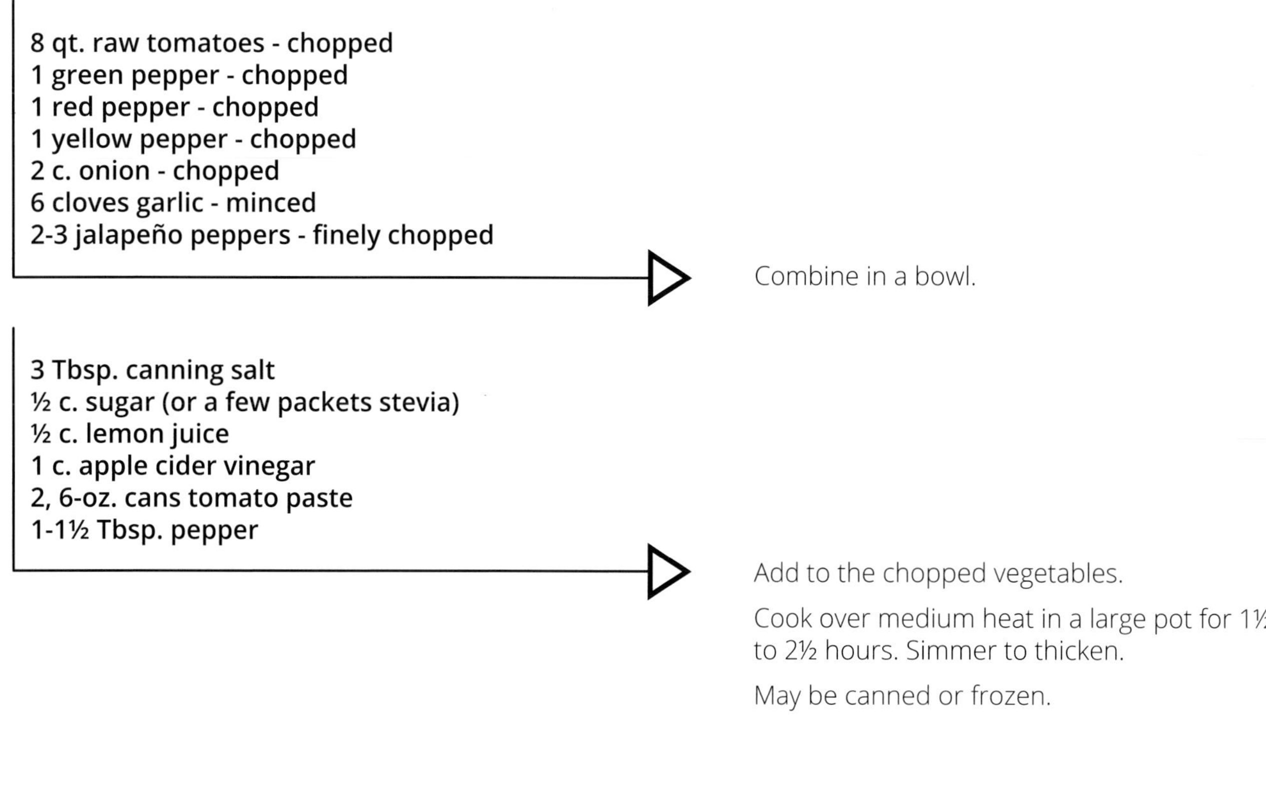

8 qt. raw tomatoes - chopped
1 green pepper - chopped
1 red pepper - chopped
1 yellow pepper - chopped
2 c. onion - chopped
6 cloves garlic - minced
2-3 jalapeño peppers - finely chopped

Combine in a bowl.

3 Tbsp. canning salt
½ c. sugar (or a few packets stevia)
½ c. lemon juice
1 c. apple cider vinegar
2, 6-oz. cans tomato paste
1-1½ Tbsp. pepper

Add to the chopped vegetables.

Cook over medium heat in a large pot for 1½ to 2½ hours. Simmer to thicken.

May be canned or frozen.

To Balance the Meal: serve over 4 oz. grilled chicken with ½ avocado and ½ c. black beans.

To make gluten free:
This meal is gluten free

To make dairy free:
This meal is dairy free

Marinades & Seasonings

Pesto Marinade
1, 8-oz. jar pre-made pesto
Juice of 1 lemon
¼ c. olive oil

Shake in an opaque container with a tight-fitting lid.

Thai Satay
1 can coconut milk
½ c. natural peanut butter
1 Tbsp. Bragg Liquid Aminos

Blend until creamy.

Rosemary
¼ c. olive oil
1 tsp. salt
½ tsp. pepper
3 Tbsp. dried rosemary
2 cloves minced garlic

Shake in an opaque container with a tight-fitting lid.

Spicy Caribbean Jerk
1 white onion
1-2 jalapeños - stems removed
1-4 habañeros or Scotch Bonnet peppers - stems removed (optional)
4 cloves garlic
1 tsp. ground cloves
1 tsp. ground nutmeg
1 tsp. ground cinnamon
¼ c. fresh lime juice
¼ c. olive oil
2 Tbsp. Bragg Liquid Aminos

Purée all ingredients in a food processor or blender.

Cajun Seasoning
2 tsp. paprika
1 tsp. sea salt
1 tsp. garlic powder
1 tsp. onion powder
¼ tsp. black pepper
¼ tsp. dried oregano leaves
¼ tsp. dried thyme

Shake all spices together in a jar with a tight-fitting lid.

Simple Salad Dressing

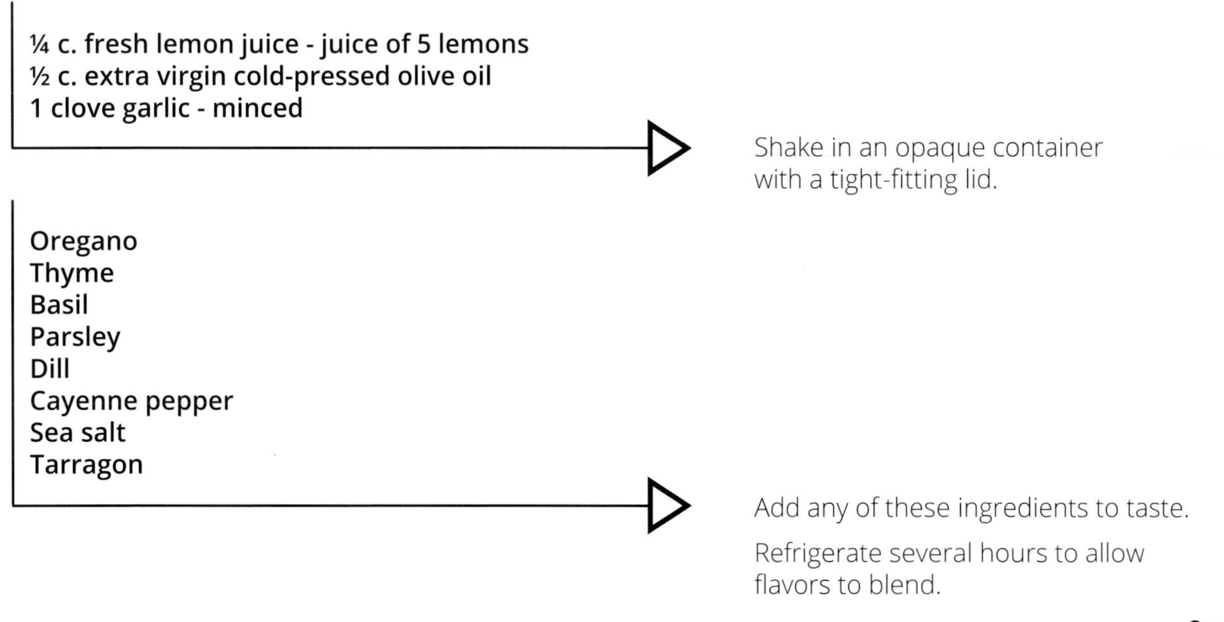

¼ c. fresh lemon juice - juice of 5 lemons
½ c. extra virgin cold-pressed olive oil
1 clove garlic - minced

Shake in an opaque container with a tight-fitting lid.

Oregano
Thyme
Basil
Parsley
Dill
Cayenne pepper
Sea salt
Tarragon

Add any of these ingredients to taste.

Refrigerate several hours to allow flavors to blend.

Serves 8

To Balance the Meal: drizzle over a large salad with 4 c. greens, 2 c. vegetables, and a 4 oz. chicken breast with ½ avocado sliced on top.

To make gluten free:
This dressing is gluten free

To make dairy free:
This dressing is dairy free

Super Simple Ranch Dressing

½ c. cold-pressed mayonnaise
½ c. sour cream
½ c. buttermilk
2 tsp. dried chives
2 tsp. dried parsley
2 tsp. dried dill
1 tsp. dried oregano
1 clove minced garlic
½ tsp. salt

Combine in a bowl.

Serves 7

To Balance the Meal: serve with a large salad and 4 oz. grass-fed steak.

To make gluten free:
This dressing is gluten free

To make dairy free:
This dressing cannot be made dairy free

Managing Diabetes the Weight & Wellness Way

I am diabetic. What will happen to my blood sugar while eating this way?

You may be surprised at how much easier it is to stabilize your blood sugar when you eat a balance of protein, healthy fats and carbohydrates five to six times each day. The Weight & Wellness Way of eating keeps insulin levels from spiking or plummeting and gives you clearer thinking and sustained energy. Healthy fats like olive oil, avocados, nuts and butter satisfy hunger and stabilize blood sugar. For that reason, we recommend eating healthy fats at every meal and snack.

Gary's success story—lost 50 pounds and reduced glucose numbers by 300 points

I have finally reduced my blood sugar numbers! They have gone from 300-400 to below 110. I truly understand how dangerous processed carbohydrates are for diabetics. The wonderful thing is that I am not hungry because I add sufficient healthy fats to every meal and snack. Still, I can't believe that I eat butter and sour cream and have lost more than 50 pounds in the last few months. I feel better now, think clearly and can enjoy playing with my grand kids.

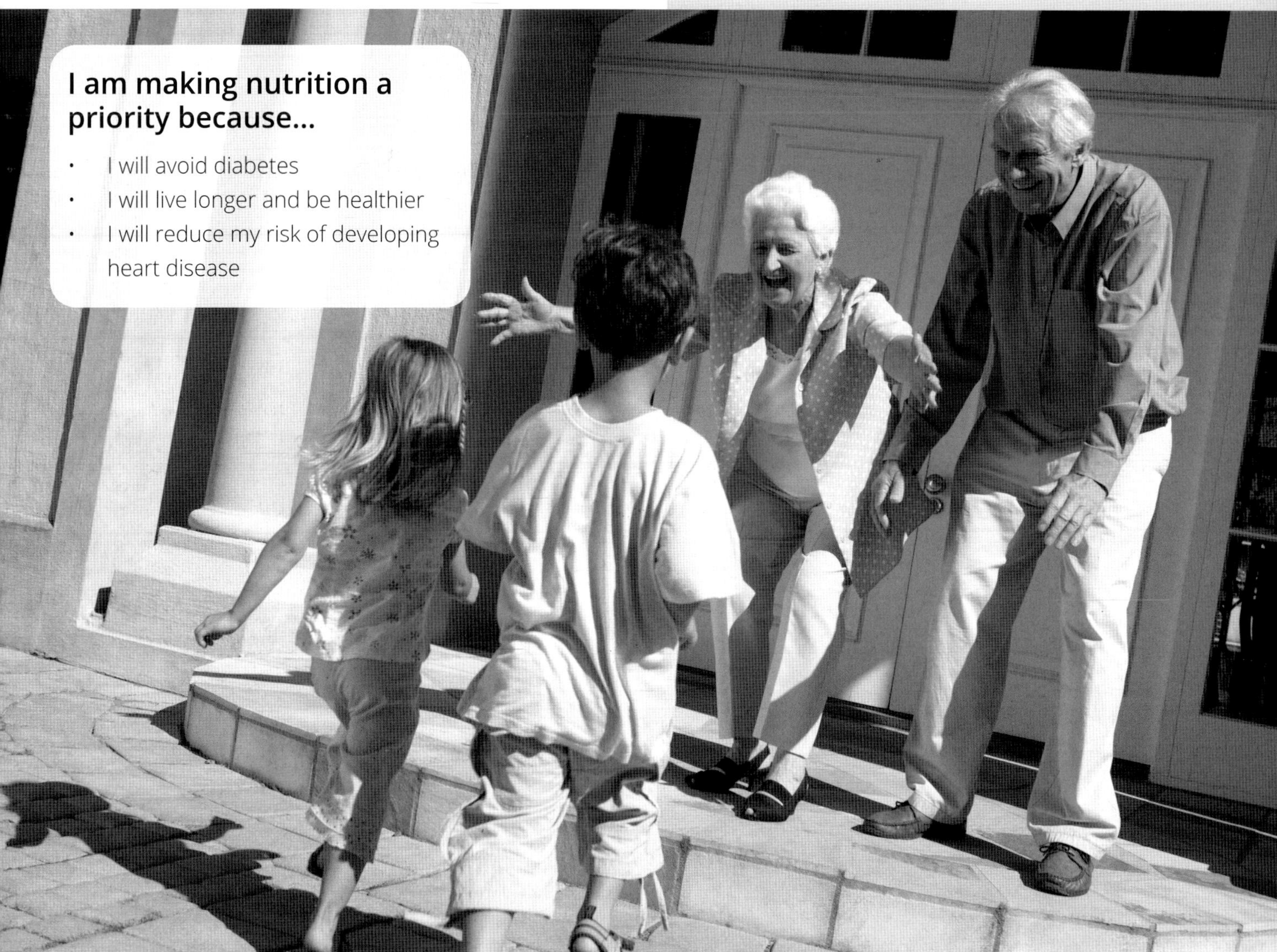

I am making nutrition a priority because...

- I will avoid diabetes
- I will live longer and be healthier
- I will reduce my risk of developing heart disease

Vegetables

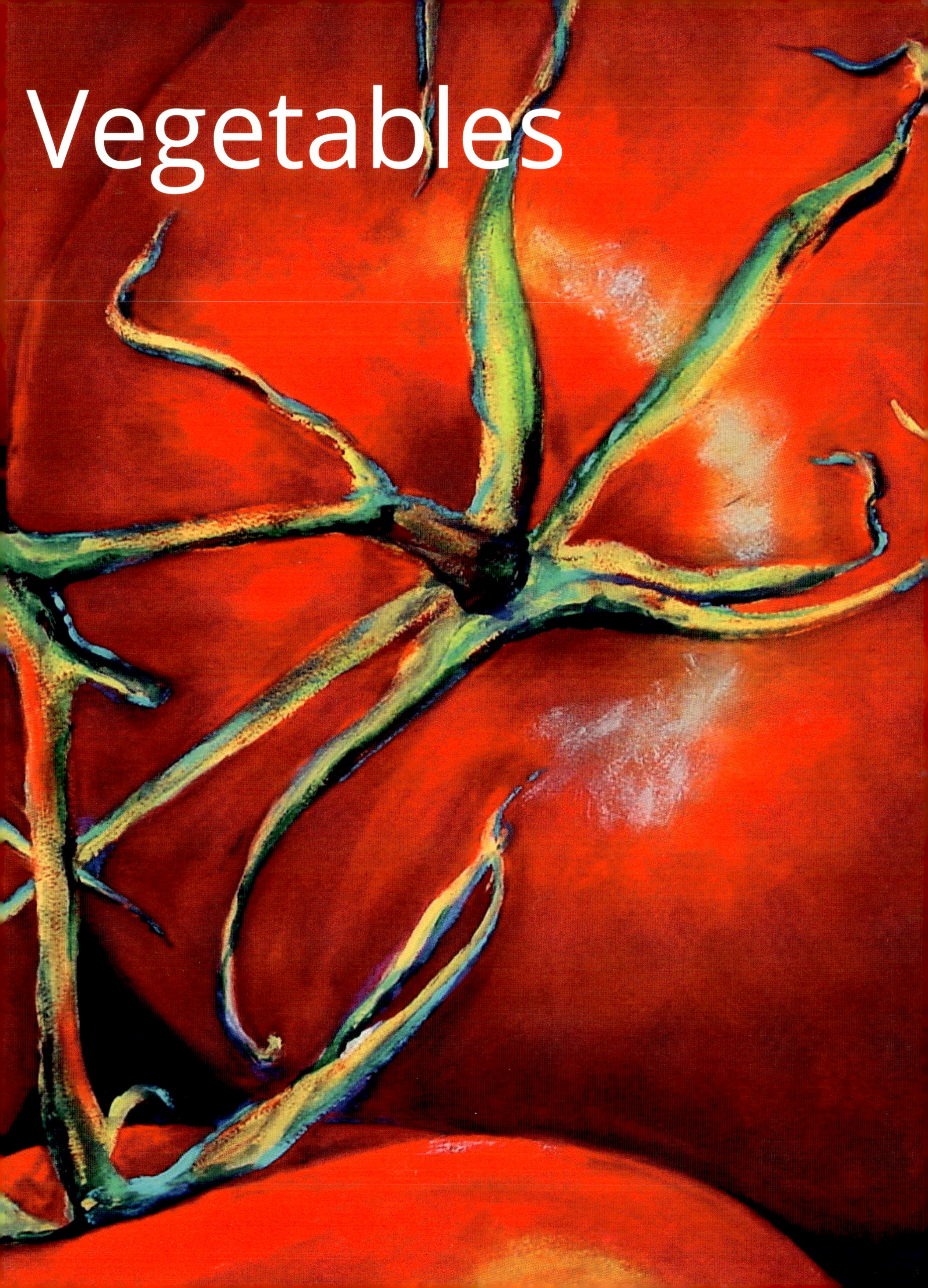

Brussels Sprouts Sauté

2 tsp. butter
2 Tbsp. olive oil
1 c. onion, chopped
4 c. Brussels sprouts - cleaned and halved
1 c. green pepper - chopped
1 c. red pepper - chopped
1 c. yellow pepper - chopped
1 tsp. salt and pepper to taste

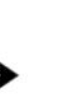

Heat a large sauté pan to medium and add butter and olive oil. Add Brussels sprouts and onions and cook for 8 minutes. Add other vegetables and sauté for about 5 minutes more. Season with salt and pepper.

Serves 4

To Balance the Meal: serve with a 4-ounce pork chop and ½ c. rice.

To make gluten free:
This meal is gluten free

To make dairy free:
Use coconut oil instead of butter

Cajun Beans

2 Tbsp. avocado or coconut oil
2 c. celery – diced
½ c. onion – chopped
1 c. green pepper – chopped
1 c. red pepper – chopped

Sauté in a 4-quart saucepan.

1 can black or pinto beans - drained and rinsed
1½ lbs. cooked chicken (or turkey) breast - cut into 1" squares
1 c. corn - fresh or frozen
1 c. broth - preservative free
1 clove garlic - minced
1 bay leaf
1 tsp. Cajun Seasonings (p.133) - to taste

Add to saucepan, bring to a boil, and then simmer for 20 minutes. Remove bay leaf.

Serves 6

To Balance the Meal: serve with 2 Tbsp. sour cream or avocado slices.

To make gluten free:
This meal is gluten free

To make dairy free:
Substitute olive oil for sour cream

Carrots and Parsnips

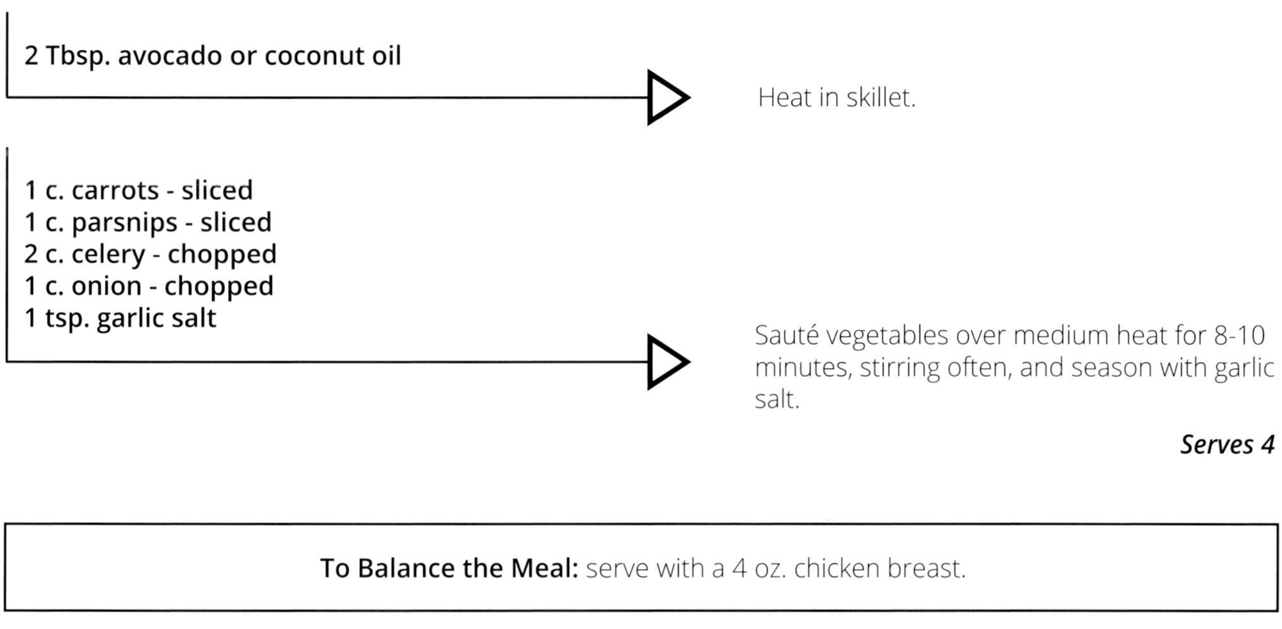

2 Tbsp. avocado or coconut oil

Heat in skillet.

1 c. carrots - sliced
1 c. parsnips - sliced
2 c. celery - chopped
1 c. onion - chopped
1 tsp. garlic salt

Sauté vegetables over medium heat for 8-10 minutes, stirring often, and season with garlic salt.

Serves 4

To Balance the Meal: serve with a 4 oz. chicken breast.

To make gluten free:
This meal is gluten free

To make dairy free:
This meal is dairy free

Collard Greens

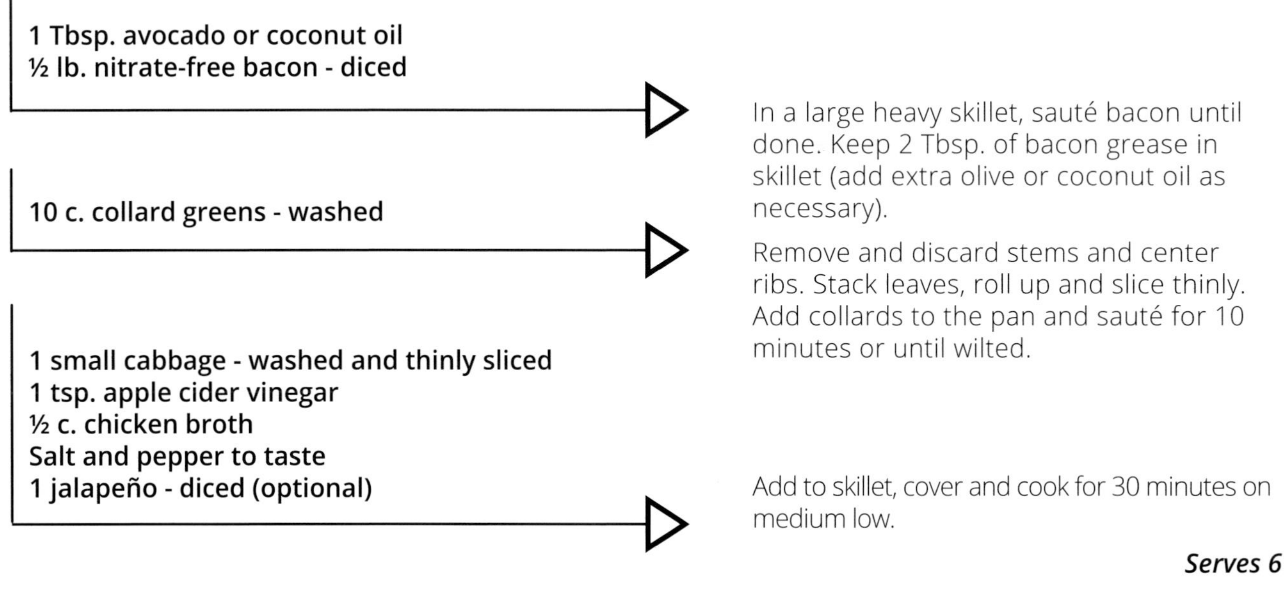

1 Tbsp. avocado or coconut oil
½ lb. nitrate-free bacon - diced

In a large heavy skillet, sauté bacon until done. Keep 2 Tbsp. of bacon grease in skillet (add extra olive or coconut oil as necessary).

10 c. collard greens - washed

Remove and discard stems and center ribs. Stack leaves, roll up and slice thinly. Add collards to the pan and sauté for 10 minutes or until wilted.

1 small cabbage - washed and thinly sliced
1 tsp. apple cider vinegar
½ c. chicken broth
Salt and pepper to taste
1 jalapeño - diced (optional)

Add to skillet, cover and cook for 30 minutes on medium low.

Serves 6

To Balance the Meal: serve with Instant Pot Citrus Pork (p.76) and Sweet Potato Wedges (p.155).

To make gluten free:
This is gluten free

To make dairy free:
This is dairy free

Grilled Summer Vegetables

2 Tbsp. avocado or coconut oil
1 med yellow onion - chopped

Heat skillet and add oil. Sauté onion until translucent, about 4 minutes.

1 clove garlic - thinly sliced
2 c. zucchini - thinly sliced
1 c. green pepper - thinly sliced
2 c. summer squash - thinly sliced
2 small Roma tomatoes - quartered
1 tsp. salt
¼ tsp. ground pepper
1 Tbsp. natural balsamic vinegar

Add garlic and cook for 1 minute.

Add the vegetables, season with salt and pepper and sauté until tender.

Finish with the vinegar and serve.

Serves 4

To Balance the Meal: serve with 4 oz. of grilled steak and ½ ear of corn on the cob.

To make gluten free:
This is gluten free

To make dairy free:
This is dairy free

Leeks, Corn and Red Pepper

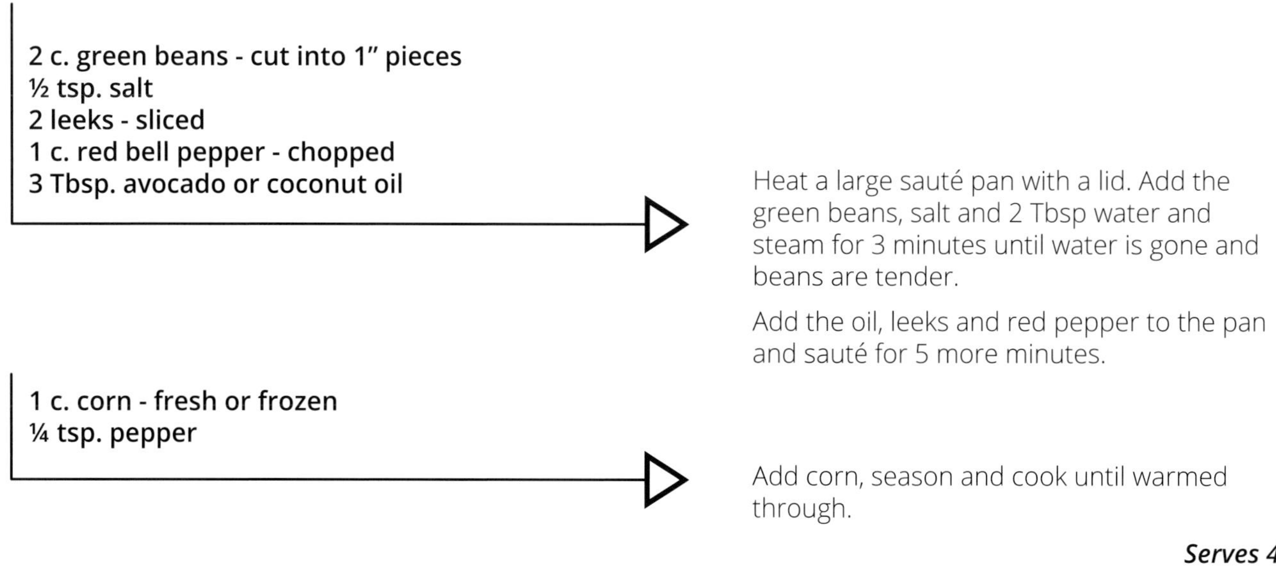

2 c. green beans - cut into 1" pieces
½ tsp. salt
2 leeks - sliced
1 c. red bell pepper - chopped
3 Tbsp. avocado or coconut oil

Heat a large sauté pan with a lid. Add the green beans, salt and 2 Tbsp water and steam for 3 minutes until water is gone and beans are tender.

Add the oil, leeks and red pepper to the pan and sauté for 5 more minutes.

1 c. corn - fresh or frozen
¼ tsp. pepper

Add corn, season and cook until warmed through.

Serves 4

To Balance the Meal: serve with a 4 oz. cooked chicken breast and ½ c. cooked quinoa.

To make gluten free:
This is gluten free

To make dairy free:
This is dairy free

Mashed Potatoes and Cauliflower

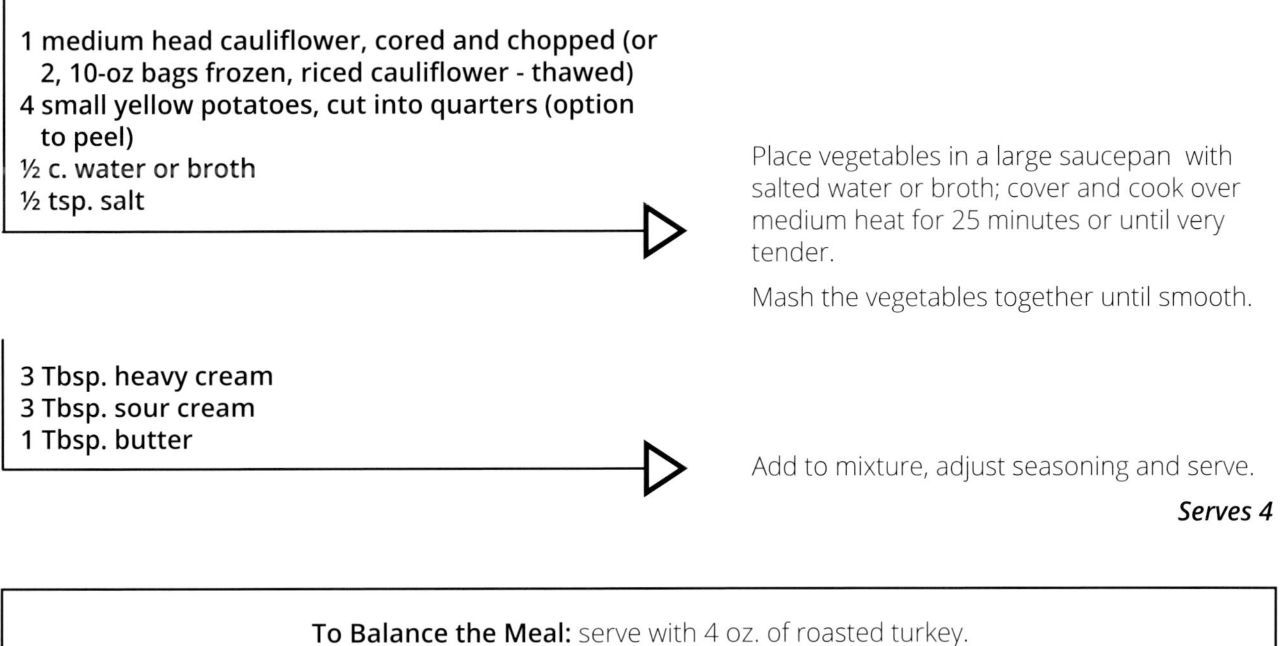

1 medium head cauliflower, cored and chopped (or 2, 10-oz bags frozen, riced cauliflower - thawed)
4 small yellow potatoes, cut into quarters (option to peel)
½ c. water or broth
½ tsp. salt

Place vegetables in a large saucepan with salted water or broth; cover and cook over medium heat for 25 minutes or until very tender.

Mash the vegetables together until smooth.

3 Tbsp. heavy cream
3 Tbsp. sour cream
1 Tbsp. butter

Add to mixture, adjust seasoning and serve.

Serves 4

To Balance the Meal: serve with 4 oz. of roasted turkey.

To make gluten free:
This meal is gluten free

To make dairy free:
Replace the heavy cream and sour cream with ¼ c. coconut milk and replace the butter with coconut oil

Oven Ratatouille

1 medium globe eggplant - cubed
2 zucchini, cut into ½" pieces
1 medium yellow onion - sliced
3 cloves garlic - thinly sliced
4 plum tomatoes - quartered
1 medium green or red bell pepper - thickly sliced
½ tsp. oregano or 1 tsp. Italian herb blend
¼ tsp. thyme
1 tsp. salt and pepper to taste
¼ c. olive oil

Preheat oven to 325°.

Combine vegetables and seasonings, add olive oil and toss well to coat.

Place all ingredients in a 3-quart casserole dish and bake uncovered for 1-1 ½ hours.

2 Tbsp. fresh basil leaves - chopped
1 Tbsp. fresh Italian parsley - chopped

Finish with fresh herbs before serving.

Serves 4

This recipe can be made as a sheet pan meal: Place vegetables onto sheet pan after tossing in bowl with oil (keeping garlic whole). Roast at 375° for 45 minutes, stir halfway through.

To Balance the Meal: serve with 4 oz. roasted chicken thighs, ½ c. brown rice and 2 tsp. butter.

To make gluten free:
This is gluten free

To make dairy free:
This is dairy free

Pan-Roasted Cabbage and Carrots

4 c. green cabbage - thinly sliced into 2" pieces
4 c. purple cabbage - thinly sliced into 2" pieces
2 c. carrots - shredded with vegetable peeler
¼ c. water or broth
1 tsp. salt
1 tsp. caraway or fennel seed
2 Tbsp. butter

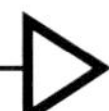

Combine in a pan, cover and simmer until tender.

Serves 4

To Balance the Meal: serve with 4 oz. baked salmon.

To make gluten free:
This is gluten free

To make dairy free:
Substitute coconut oil for butter

Fact *vs.* **Fiction**

Fiction	Fact
Butter is fattening, so I use margarine or another soft spread instead.	A tablespoon of butter has 14 grams of fat, the same amount as a tablespoon of margarine. The fat in butter activates metabolism; while the fat in margarine, a damaged fat, slows metabolism.

Parmesan Brussels Sprouts

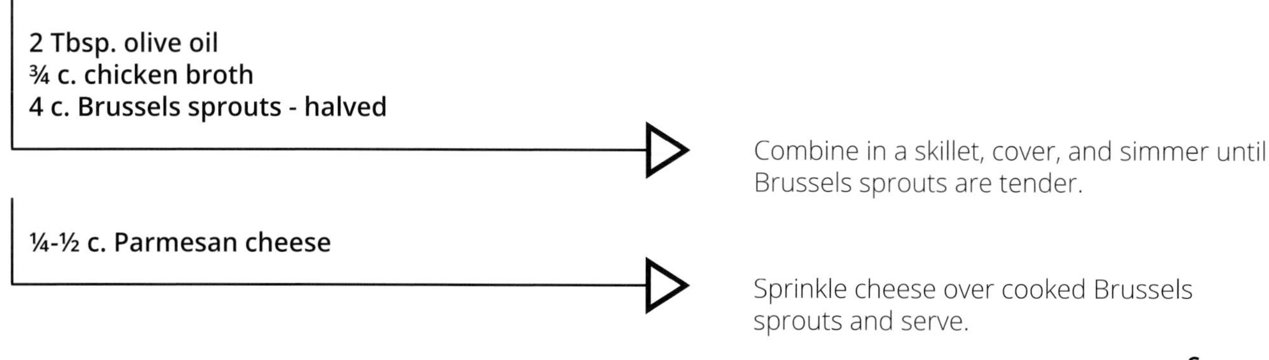

2 Tbsp. olive oil
¾ c. chicken broth
4 c. Brussels sprouts - halved

Combine in a skillet, cover, and simmer until Brussels sprouts are tender.

¼-½ c. Parmesan cheese

Sprinkle cheese over cooked Brussels sprouts and serve.

Serves 4

To Balance the Meal: serve with 4 oz. chicken breast and ½ c. butternut squash topped with 1-2 tsp. butter.

To make gluten free:
This meal is gluten free

To make dairy free:
This dish cannot be made dairy free

Roasted Asparagus

1 lb. asparagus - washed and trimmed
2 tsp. olive oil
1 tsp. lemon juice
1 tsp. sea salt

Preheat oven to 375º.

Coat asparagus in olive oil and lemon juice and sprinkle on salt.

Place on baking sheet and cook in upper third of oven for 10-12 minutes or until spears are tender when poked with the tip of a knife.

Serves 4

To Balance the Meal: serve with a 4 oz. steak, ½ c. sweet potato and 1 tsp. butter.

To make gluten free:
This dish is gluten free

To make dairy free:
Substitute coconut oil for butter

Roasted Autumn Vegetables

2 c. winter squash - cubed
4 c. Brussels sprouts - cut in half
4 c. cauliflower - cut into bite-size pieces
2 c. red bell pepper - thinly sliced
2 Tbsp. avocado oil
½ tsp. salt
¼ tsp. pepper

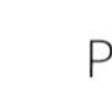

Preheat oven to 350°.

Toss vegetables in avocado oil and seasonings. Spread on a 13" x 9" baking sheet or dish. Bake for about 30 minutes. Flip vegetables over halfway through baking.

Serves 4

To Balance the Meal: serve with a 4 oz. chicken breast.

To make gluten free:
This is gluten free

To make dairy free:
This is dairy free

Roasted Parsnips

2 c. parsnips - cleaned and sliced into ½" pieces
¼ tsp. salt
3 Tbsp. avocado or coconut oil - melted

Preheat oven to 400º.

Line sheet pan with parchment paper.

Add vegetables and oil to sheet pan and mix. Roast for 20 minutes.

Serves 4

To Balance the Meal: serve with 4 oz. turkey burger and 2 c. green beans.

To make gluten free:
This is gluten free

To make dairy free:
This is dairy free

Sheetpan Eggplant

1½ Tbsp. avocado oil
1 c. yellow onion - thickly sliced
2 red peppers - cored/seeded and thickly sliced
6 c. eggplant - diced (about one large eggplant)
2 cloves garlic - whole
1 tsp. salt and pepper to taste

Preheat oven to 400°

In a large bowl, mix the vegetables with the avocado oil and season with salt and pepper.

Roast in top third of oven for 25-30 minutes until golden brown.

1 c. fresh basil (chopped)
Dash of cayenne pepper
Sea salt to taste

Remove vegetables to serving platter. With the back of a fork, mash the roasted garlic and toss with remaining ingredients.

Serves 4

To Balance the Meal: divide side dish into four servings and serve with 4 oz. salmon or steak and ½ c. cooked brown rice.

To make gluten free:
This meal is gluten free

To make dairy free:
This meal is dairy free

Summer Vegetables

2 Tbsp. avocado or coconut oil
½ c. onion - chopped
1 c. red potatoes - chopped

Sauté in a skillet for 10 minutes over medium heat.

1 c. zucchini - sliced
½ c. green pepper - sliced
1 c. summer squash - sliced
2 c. tomato - cut into wedges,
or cherry tomatoes - cut in half
½ c. green beans - trimmed
¼ tsp. ground pepper
1 clove garlic - minced
2 Tbsp. natural balsamic vinegar
1 tsp. Dijon mustard

Add and cook until tender.

Serves 2

To Balance the Meal: serve with a 4 oz. meat patty.

To make gluten free:
This dish is gluten free

To make dairy free:
This dish is dairy free

Sweet Potato Mash

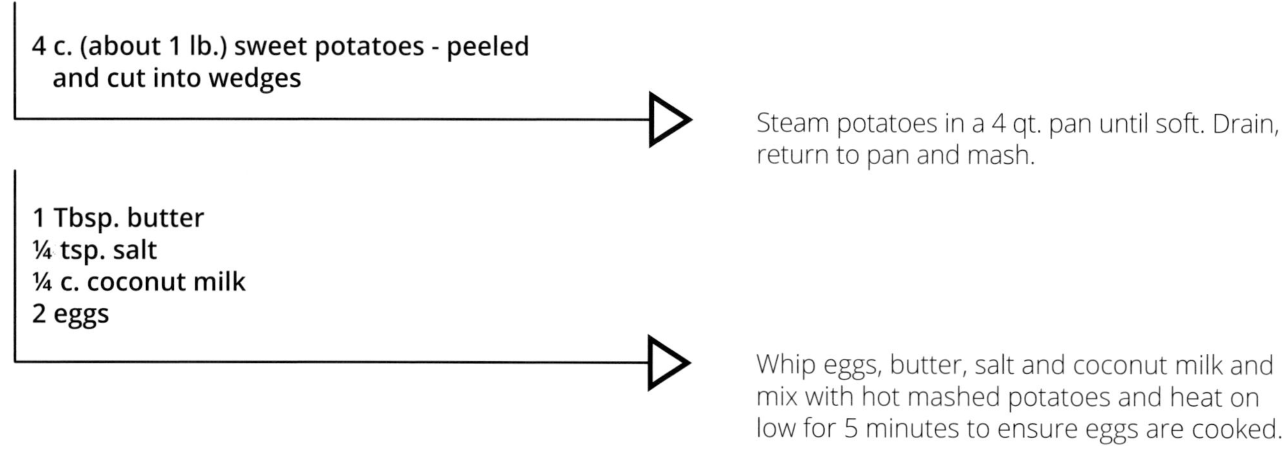

4 c. (about 1 lb.) sweet potatoes - peeled and cut into wedges

Steam potatoes in a 4 qt. pan until soft. Drain, return to pan and mash.

1 Tbsp. butter
¼ tsp. salt
¼ c. coconut milk
2 eggs

Whip eggs, butter, salt and coconut milk and mix with hot mashed potatoes and heat on low for 5 minutes to ensure eggs are cooked.

Serves 6

To Balance the Meal: serve with Dijon Crockpot Pork Chops (p.75) and 1-2 c. green beans.

To make gluten free:
This is gluten free

To make dairy free:
Substitute coconut oil for butter

Sweet Potato Wedges

2 Tbsp. avocado oil
2 medium sweet potatoes or yams - cut into wedges
1 tsp. garlic salt
1-2 tsp. dried rosemary

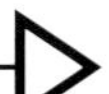

Preheat oven to 400º.

Coat wedges with avocado oil and sprinkle with seasonings.

Place on parchment-lined baking sheet and cook for 18-25 minutes, turning occasionally.

Serves 4

To Balance the Meal: serve with a 4 oz. beef patty and 1 c. green beans.

To make gluten free:
This dish is gluten free

To make dairy free:
This dish is dairy free

Zucchini Sauté

1 Tbsp. avocado or coconut oil
2 c. onion, diced
6 c. zucchini, diced
4 c. cherry tomatoes (halved)
¼ c. almond meal
½ tsp. salt

Heat a large sauté pan and add butter and olive oil.

Sauté onions for 3 minutes then add zucchini and salt and cook for 5 minutes more.

Add the tomatoes and continue cooking until they have released their juices; 3-4 minutes.

Stir in the almond meal, adjust the seasoning and serve.

.

Serves 4

To Balance the Meal: serve with 4 oz. beef patty and 1 c. green beans.

To make gluten free:
This dish is gluten free

To make dairy free:
This dish is dairy free

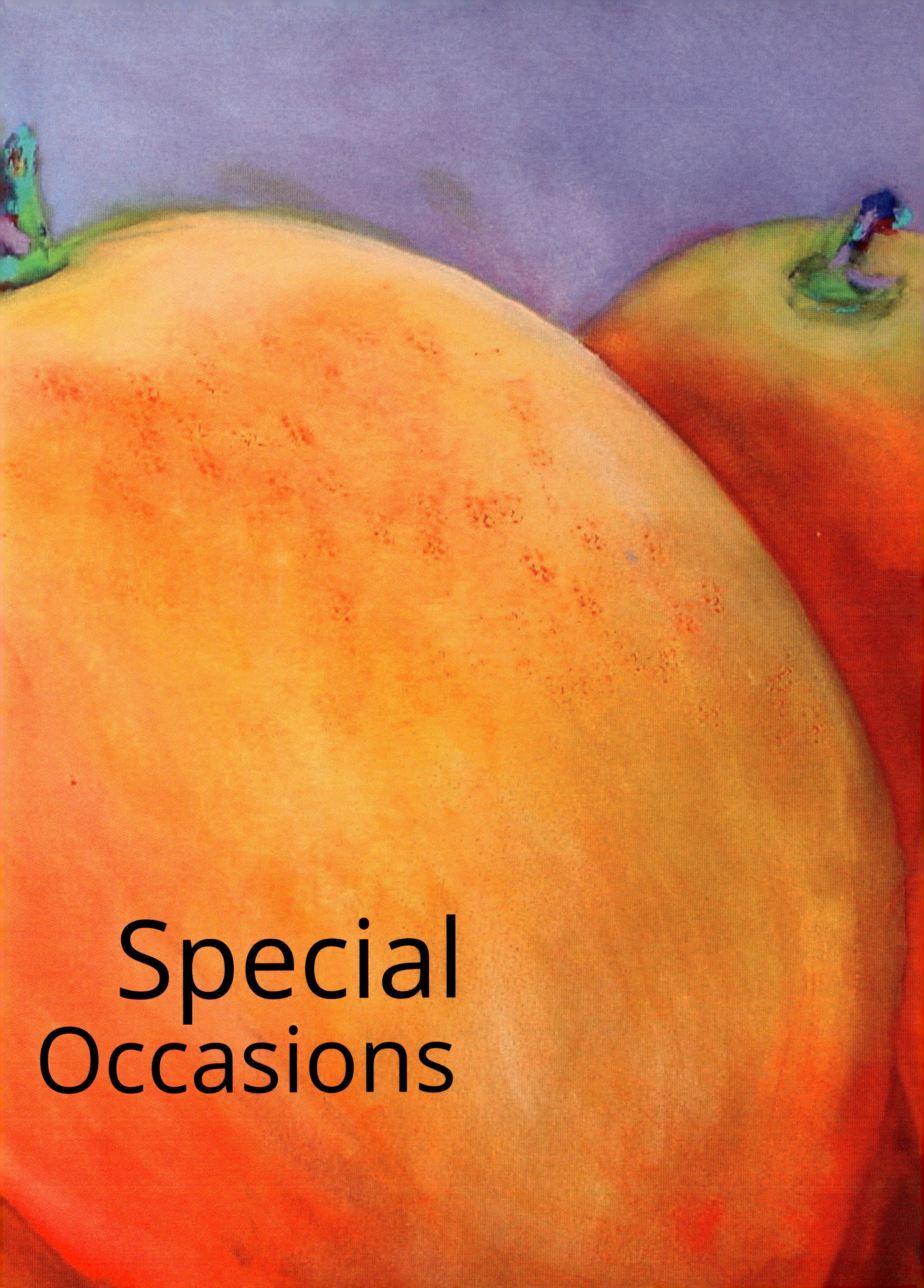
Special
Occasions

Apple Crisp

2 medium apples
2 Tbsp. lemon juice
1 Tbsp. pure maple syrup

Preheat oven to 350º.

Peel and cut apples into thin slices. Mix in lemon juice and maple syrup. Place in a baking dish.

¼ c. rolled oats
¼ c. almond flour
1 Tbsp. brown sugar
½ tsp. cinnamon
¼ tsp. nutmeg
¼ tsp. salt
1 Tbsp. cold butter - cut into small pieces

Mix with a fork until evenly combined. Sprinkle over apples. Bake for 25-30 minutes until golden brown. Cool for 10 minutes before serving.

Serves 4

To Balance the Meal: top with a dollop of freshly whipped cream and serve as dessert after a balanced meal.

To make gluten free:
This meal is gluten free

To make dairy free:
Substitute coconut oil for butter and top with whipped coconut cream

Berry-Nut Freezer Bars

Crust:
3 Tbsp. butter - room temperature
1 Tbsp. pure maple syrup
¼ tsp. salt
1 c. almond meal
½ c. coconut flour

Preheat oven to 350°. Lightly grease a 9″ x 9" pan.

Using a fork or pastry blender, mix butter, maple syrup and salt into the flours until it forms small pieces. Mixture will be very crumbly.

Press into the bottom of the pan. Bake for 8 - 10 minutes. Remove from oven and cool.

1 c. raw cashews or macadamia nuts

Soak nuts in cool water for 4 hours. Drain well but do not dry.

Place nuts in a food processor and pulse until finely chopped but not puréed.

Juice of ½ lime or lemon
¼ c. canned coconut milk
3 Tbsp. pure maple syrup
¼ c. coconut oil - melted
1 tsp. vanilla extract

Add ingredients to the chopped nuts in the food processor, blend and spread batter over the crust.

1 c. blueberries, strawberries or raspberries
2/3 c. canned coconut milk

Place berries and coconut milk into the food processor and puree (leave a couple berries out for garnish). Pour over the top of the nut batter.

Freeze for two hours or more.

Allow to thaw on the counter for 45 minutes before cutting. Store leftovers in the freezer.

Serves 16

To Balance the Meal: serve as a dessert after a balanced meal.

To make gluten free:
This dessert is gluten free

To make dairy free:
Substitute coconut oil for butter

Blueberry Fruit Glaze

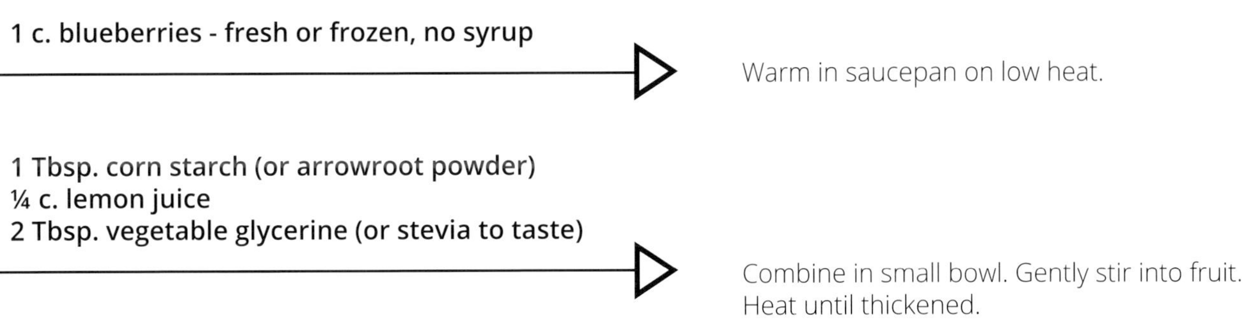

1 c. blueberries - fresh or frozen, no syrup

Warm in saucepan on low heat.

1 Tbsp. corn starch (or arrowroot powder)
¼ c. lemon juice
2 Tbsp. vegetable glycerine (or stevia to taste)

Combine in small bowl. Gently stir into fruit. Heat until thickened.

Serves 2

To Balance the Snack: stir ½ of the glaze and ½ scoop protein powder into ½ c. plain yogurt and top with 2 Tbsp. slivered almonds.

To make gluten free:
This snack is gluten free

To make dairy free:
This snack cannot be made dairy free

Peach Crisp

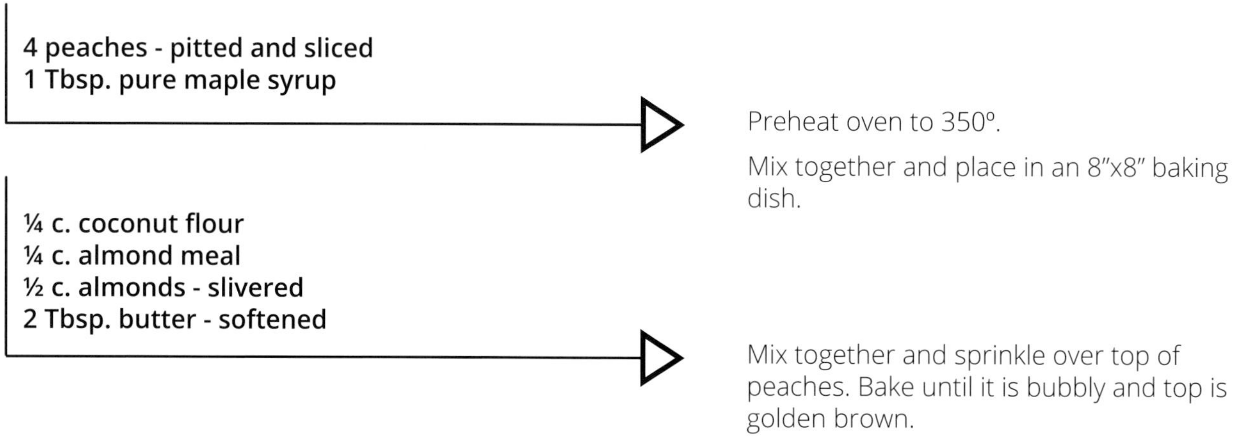

4 peaches - pitted and sliced
1 Tbsp. pure maple syrup

Preheat oven to 350º.

Mix together and place in an 8"x8" baking dish.

¼ c. coconut flour
¼ c. almond meal
½ c. almonds - slivered
2 Tbsp. butter - softened

Mix together and sprinkle over top of peaches. Bake until it is bubbly and top is golden brown.

Serves 4

To Balance the Meal: top with a dollop of freshly whipped cream and serve as a dessert after a balanced meal.

To make gluten free:
This dessert is gluten free

To make dairy free:
Substitute coconut oil for butter and top with whipped coconut cream

Pumpkin Cheesecake Bars

Crust:
3 Tbsp. butter - room temperature
1 c. almond meal
½ c. coconut flour
2 Tbsp. pure maple syrup

Preheat oven to 325°. Lightly grease a 9″ x 9" pan.

Using a fork or pastry blender, mix butter and maple syrup into the flours until it forms small balls and pieces. Mixture will be very crumbly.

Pat mixture into the bottom of pan. Bake for 7-10 minutes. Remove from the oven and cool.

16 oz. cream cheese - room temperature
15 oz. pumpkin purée
¼ c. pure maple syrup
1 tsp. vanilla
1 tsp. cinnamon
¼ tsp. ground cloves
¼ tsp. nutmeg
½ tsp. ground ginger
½ tsp. salt

Whip cream cheese on medium speed for one minute.

Add pumpkin purée, maple syrup, vanilla and spices, continue to beat for 30 seconds.

3 eggs

Add eggs one at a time until just incorporated into batter.

Pour over baked pie crust.

Create a water bath by placing ½-1" of water in a roasting pan or pan large enough to hold the 9″x9" pan. Make sure the water level is below the top edge of the pan.

Place the 9″x9″ into the water bath and bake 60 minutes, until the cheesecake has set, but still jiggles.

Turn off the oven and crack the oven door open. Allow cheesecake to rest in the oven 15-30 minutes.

Remove from oven and run a knife around the edge of the pan. Allow to cool completely before slicing.

Serves 16

To Balance the Meal: serve as a dessert after a balanced meal.

To make gluten free:
This dessert is gluten free

To make dairy free:
This dessert cannot be made dairy free

Tropical Fruit Salad

1 medium banana - sliced
1 orange - peeled and cut into chunks
1 c. fresh or canned pineapple chunks - packed in water and drained
1 c. whole strawberries - cut in half
¼ c. unsweetened dried flaked coconut
Juice of 1 lime

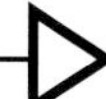

Combine all ingredients in a bowl and refrigerate 1 hour.

Serves 6

To Balance the Meal: serve with Egg Bake (p. 38).

To make gluten free:
This is gluten free

To make dairy free:
This is dairy free

Fact *VS.* **Fiction**

Fiction	Fact
I drink juice, which is healthy, instead of soda.	A glass of juice contains 17 tsp. of sugar, the same amount as a can of soda.

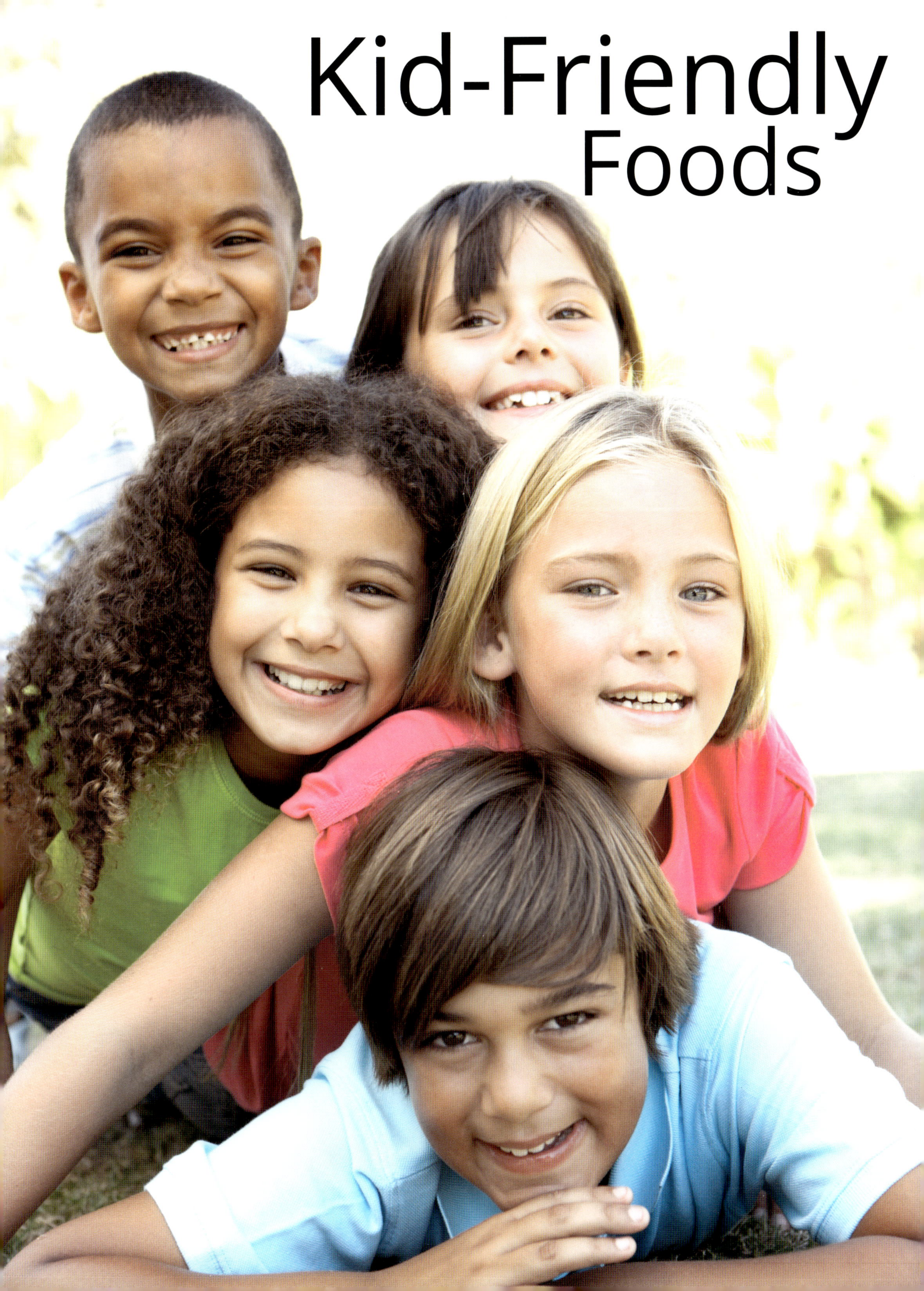
Kid-Friendly
Foods

5 Balanced Kid Lunches

Protein	Carbs	Fats	Yum
Wild Rice Meatballs (p. 57)	*Sweet Potato Wedges (p. 155)*	Olives	Wild Rice Meatballs with Sweet Potato Wedges and olives
Kabobs	***Carrots & Parsnips (p. 141),*** cherry tomatoes, green pepper	Butter	Steak, cherry tomatoes, green pepper kabobs, Carrots & Parsnips cooked in butter
Chicken or Turkey Nuggets (p. 86)	Vegetable sticks, banana	Almond butter	Chicken or Turkey Nuggets and vegetable sticks with banana and almond butter
Chili (p. 52)	Apple	Cream cheese	Chili, apple slices with cream cheese
Chicken Quesadilla	Tortilla, black beans, salsa, mixed berries	Sour cream, cheese	A chicken, cheese and black bean quesadilla made with a brown rice tortilla, topped with salsa and sour cream, with a side of mixed berries

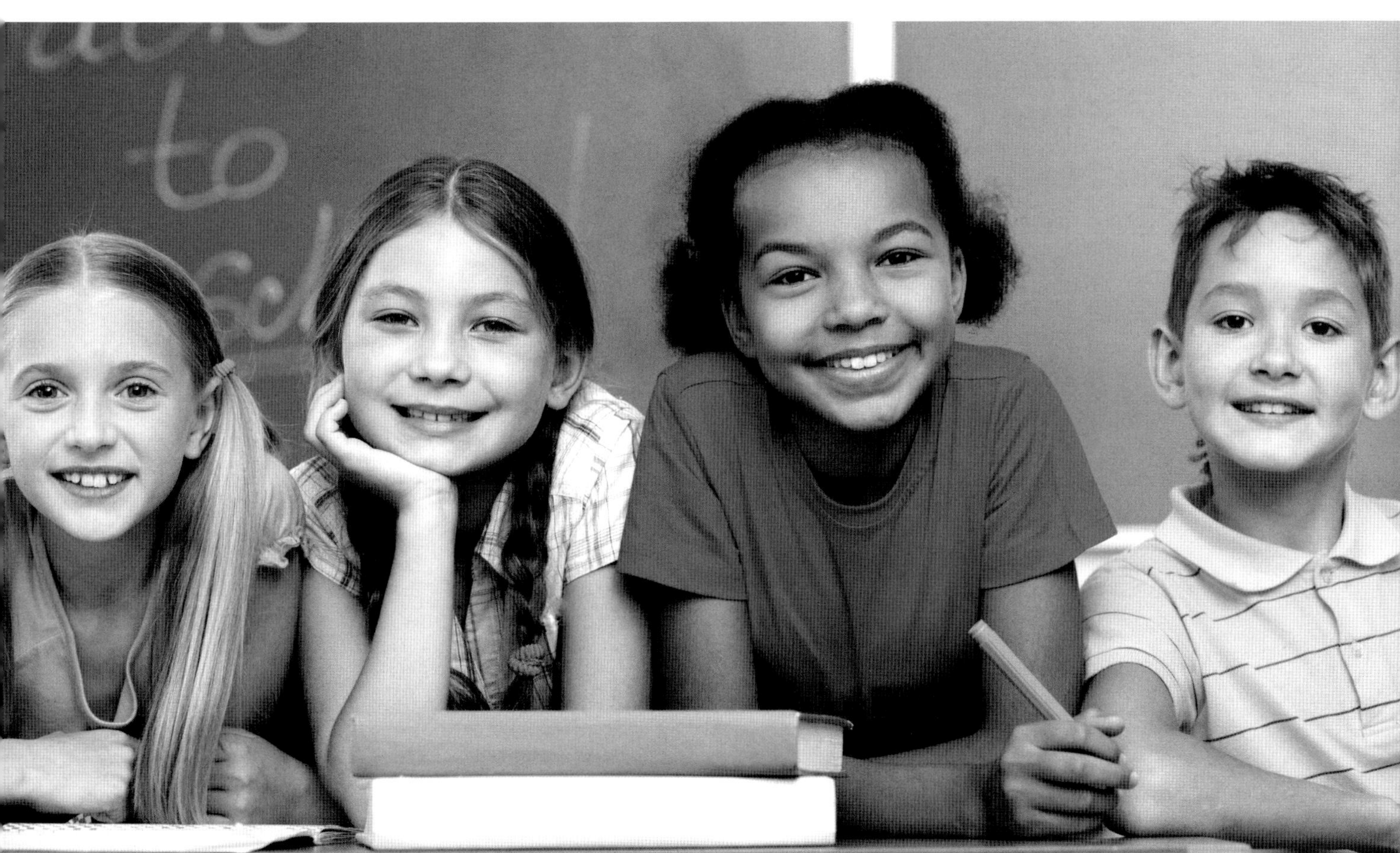

Getting Your Kids to Eat Healthier

Kids like to be part of the process, from start to finish. We have several suggestions for helping them connect with food from shopping to cooking to eating.

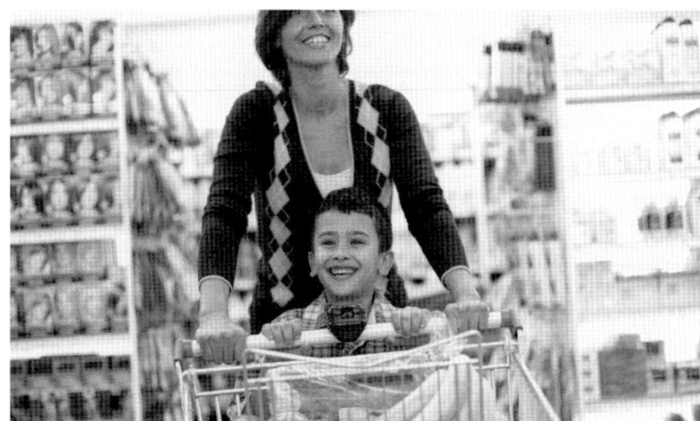

Take kids shopping and have them name vegetables they recognize and find new vegetables to try each shopping trip. Ask someone in the produce section how to prepare and serve it.

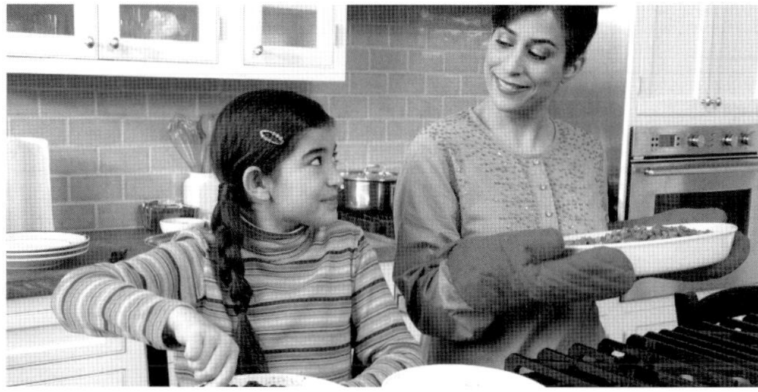

Ask kids to help prepare both raw and cooked vegetables. Find a favorite dip, like our Super Simple Ranch Dressing (p. 135) for snacking with veggies. Experiment with ways to cook veggies from sautéing to steaming and using in other dishes.

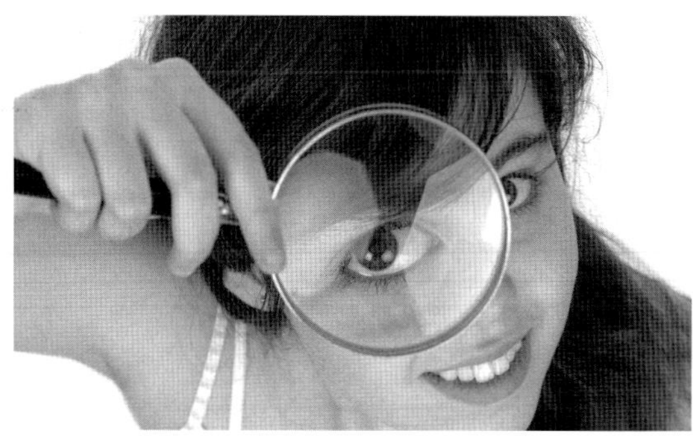

Discuss "detective label reading" and teach kids how to choose the best products without bad fats (hydrogenated or partially hydrogenated oils), added sugars, artificial sweeteners and preservatives.

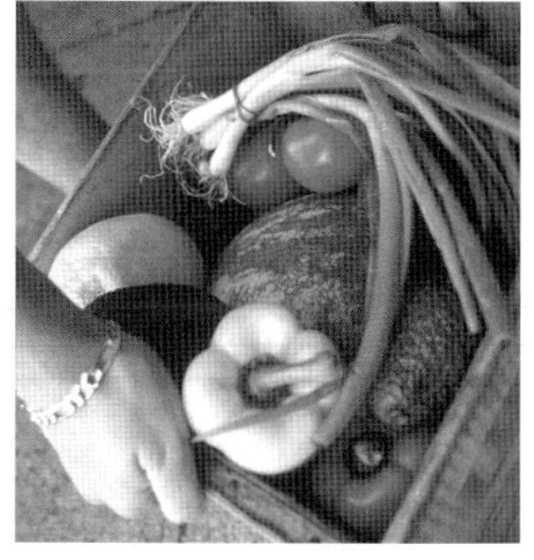

Choose a variety of vegetables, incorporating a mix of colors each time you shop.

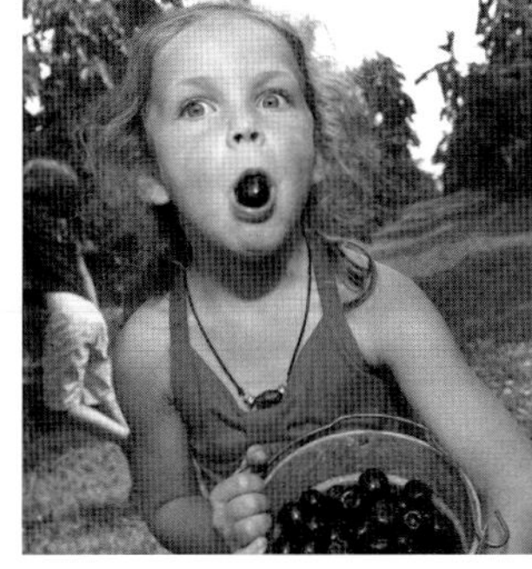

Pick your own berries, apples, pumpkins, etc. at area farms.

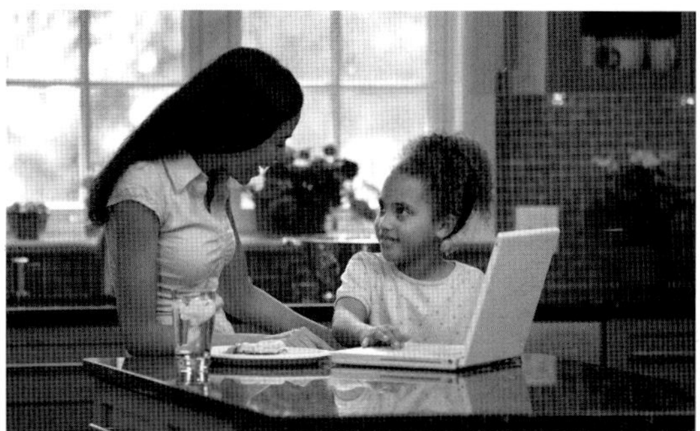

Have kids research foods and learn where different foods are grown. Look for new recipes on the Internet or in cookbooks and let children select a recipe that you can prepare together.

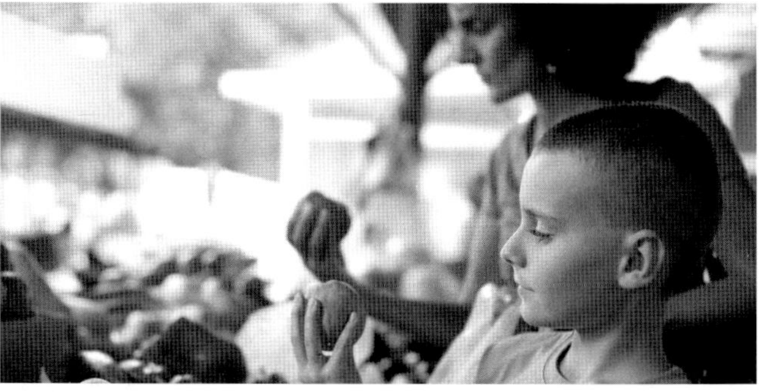

Take a family trip to the farmer's market. Meet the farmers; see how fresh produce looks at the market from Brussels sprout trees to eggplants. Let kids ask questions and help select the trays of broccoli or carrots.

Kid-Friendly Recipes

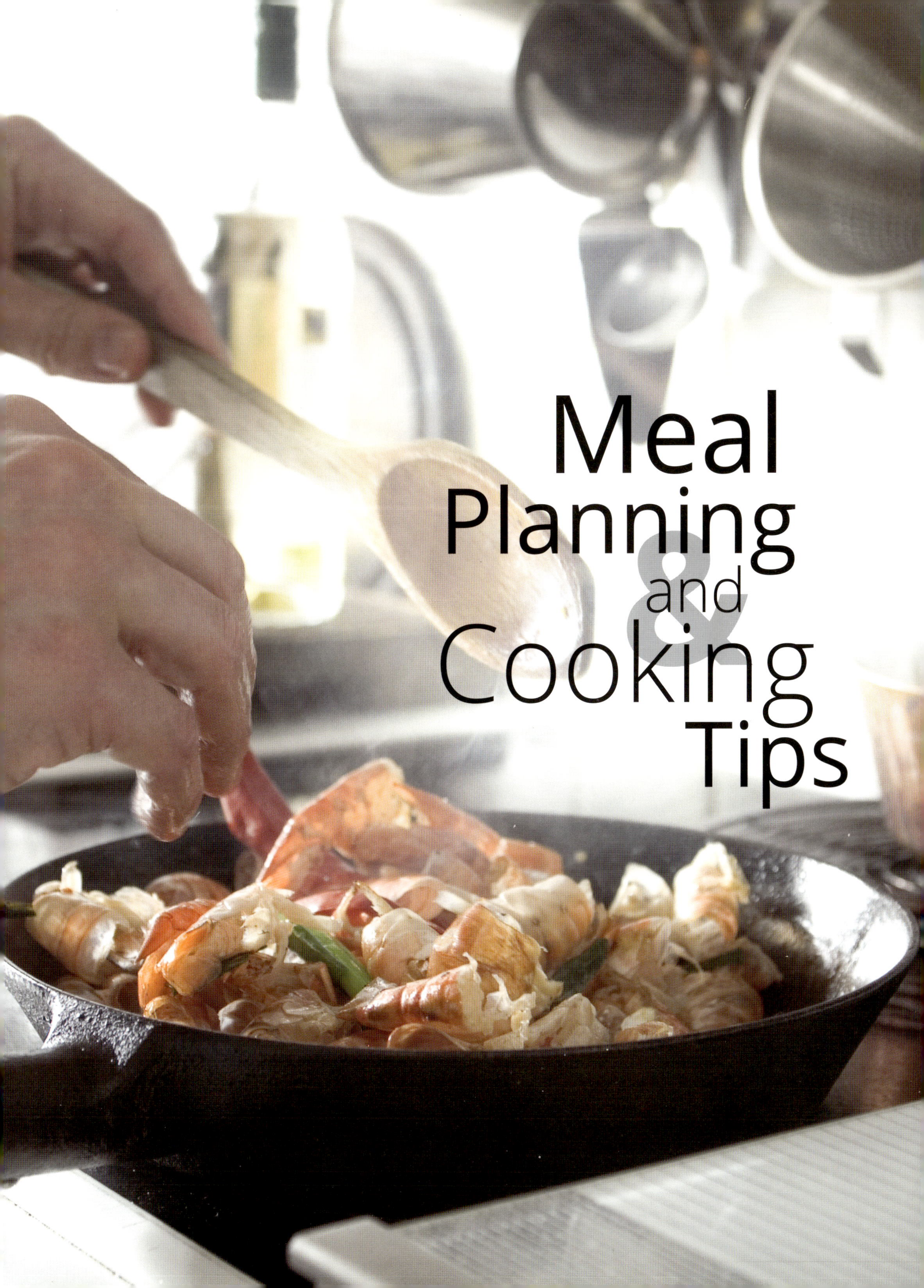

Meal Planning and Cooking Tips

7 Days of Balanced Meals and Snacks

Breakfast	Omelet (2 eggs) 1 oz. Parmesan cheese ¼ c. onion ½ c. red pepper ¼ c. green pepper ¼ c. celery ½ sweet potato 1 Tbsp. butter Top with salsa	***(2) Turkey Breakfast Sausages (p. 42)*** 12 spears asparagus ½ sweet potato 2 Tbsp. coconut oil	***Egg Bake (p. 38)*** ½ c. cantaloupe	Cottage cheese Slice of rye toast 2 Tbsp. almond butter	2 hard boiled eggs 1 sliced apple 2 Tbsp. nut butter	***Blueberry Muffin (p. 33)*** 1 oz. nitrate-free deli ham 1 Tbsp. cream cheese	Fried eggs (2) 1 c. cooked broccoli 1 sliced tomato (raw) 1 sliced cucumber (raw) ½ avocado 1 Tbsp. butter
Lunch	Taco Salad: 4 oz. meat ½ c. tomatoes ½ c. peppers ½ c. black beans 2 Tbsp. chopped onion 3 c. lettuce 1 Tbsp. sour cream ¼ c. salsa (optional) 2 Tbsp. guacamole	***Chicken Wild Rice Soup (p. 106)*** Celery and carrot sticks with almond butter	4 oz. pork tenderloin *1 c.* ***Zucchini Sauté (p. 156)*** ½ c. blueberries	***Chili (p. 52)*** Celery and carrot sticks *1 Tbsp. Super* ***Simple Ranch Dressing (p. 135)***	Roasted chicken thighs Brussels sprouts ½ c. brown or wild rice	***Easy Salmon Salad (p. 119)*** Mary's Gone Crackers	4½ oz. turkey patty 1 c. ***Crunchy Broccoli Salad (p. 116)*** 2 Wasa Light Rye crackers
Snack	(¾ c.) ***Quinoa Salad with Turkey (p. 122)***	1 chicken leg Carrot and celery sticks ¼ c. hummus	Turkey roll-up: 1-2 slices nitrate-free turkey 1 Tbsp. regular cream cheese Spread cream cheese on turkey and roll up. 1 small orange	Smoked salmon (2 oz.) 1 Tbsp. cream cheese ½ slice whole grain, 100% rye bread	Tuna salad (¼ c.) Wasa, Ryvita or gluten free cracker	Sliced steak (1-2 oz.) 1 small apple 6 - 10 olives	Nitrate-free ham (2 oz.) 1 Tbsp. cream cheese ½ brown rice tortilla
Dinner	4 oz. flank steak ½ yam 1 Tbsp. butter Small green salad with olive oil dressing	Salmon ***Brussels Sprouts Sauté (p. 139)*** ***Roasted Parsnips (p. 151)***	***Wild Rice Meatballs (p. 57)*** Tossed spinach salad ½ c. ***Carrots and Parsnips (p. 141)***	***Confetti Turkey Loaf (p. 79)*** ***Avocado & Tomato Chutney (p. 113)*** ½ sweet potato	***Instant Pot Citrus Pork (p. 76)*** ½ c. ***Sweet Potato Wedges (p. 155)*** 1 c. fresh green beans	***Shepherd's Pie (51)***	***Deep Dish Pizza Pie (p. 54)***
Bedtime Snack	Apple slices with 1 Tbsp. cream cheese or almond butter	Avocado pudding: mash together ½ avocado with ½ banana	Apple or pear slices sautéed in butter with walnuts, cinnamon and nutmeg, topped with 2 Tbsp. heavy cream or coconut milk or ½ c. whipped cream	½ c. berries, topped with 2 Tbsp. heavy cream or coconut milk or ½ c. whipped cream	Celery sticks with 2 Tbsp. cream cheese	¼ c. canned coconut milk with ½ scoop chocolate Key Greens & Fruits	½ c. sweet potatoes with 2 tsp. butter

Planning Balanced Meals

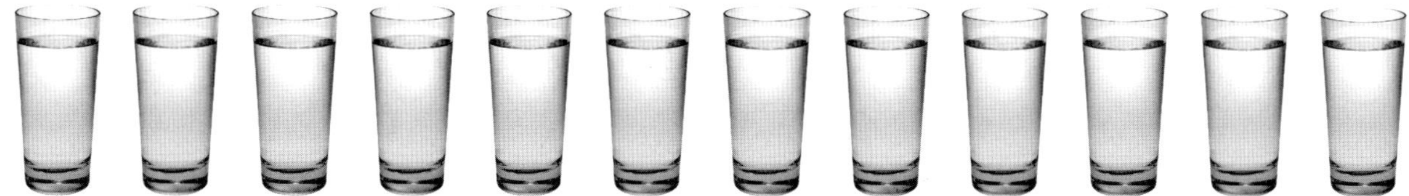

BREAKFAST

Protein ☐ ______

Carbohydrate ☐ ______

Fat ☐ ______

SNACK

Protein ☐ ______

Carbohydrate ☐ ______

Fat ☐ ______

LUNCH

Protein ☐ ______

Carbohydrate ☐ ______

Fat ☐ ______

SNACK

Protein ☐ ______

Carbohydrate ☐ ______

Fat ☐ ______

DINNER

Protein ☐ ______

Carbohydrate ☐ ______

Fat ☐ ______

SNACK

Carbohydrate ☐ ______

Fat ☐ ______

Grilling Tips

Charcoal or gas?

Both types of grilling offer perks: gas is quick but charcoal delivers great flavor. If you're using charcoal, we recommend using natural lump hardwood charcoal instead of briquettes for fuel. Avoid lighting charcoal with lighter fluid, instead use a charcoal chimney or get an electric charcoal lighter.

Prepare your meat

Marinating meat increases it's tenderness and flavor. If you're not using a marinade, be sure to season your meat generously. Allow meat to come to room temperature before putting it on the grill.

Prepare your grill

Light the grill and allow it to heat up to 400-500º. Use a wire brush to scrape the grate clean. You may want to grease the grill with a paper towel soaked in coconut oil to prevent sticking, especially when grilling fish.

Throw it on

Put the meat on the hot grill. Allow it to sear for a minute then flip it over and sear for a minute on the other side. Turn the heat down, between 200-300º. Cooking at this lower temperature prevents charring and flare ups. Cook until meat is cooked through.

Give it a rest

Remove the meat from the grill and allow it to rest on a plate for 10-15 minutes. This lets the meat finish cooking and the juices to re-absorb into the meat. After the rest, cut the meat at a diagonal across the grain.

Grilling veggies

Toss vegetables in a bowl with avocado or coconut oil and seasoning. Use a grill basket or grill pan when grilling veggies and fish to avoid sacrificing your delicious food to the grill gods. Grill on both sides until tender, but still crispy.

Tips for Cooking Grass-Fed Meat

- Turn down the heat. Grass-fed meat is lower in fat and can become tough when cooked at higher temperatures.
- Check the temperature. We recommend using a meat thermometer to avoid overcooking the meat.
- Cook low and slow. Our favorite way to cook grass-fed meat is at temperatures below 200º for several hours. Super-slow roasting or grilling keeps the meat tender, juicy and flavorful.
- Season lightly. To enjoy the true flavor of grass-fed meat, be careful not to over-season it.

Nine Slow Cooker Tips

We love using slow cookers year-round because they are great time-savers, and there's nothing better than arriving home at the end of a long day and having a hot meal ready to eat.

Check out these slow cooker tips and recipes to make the most out of your slow cooker meals:

1. When entertaining holiday guests, it is helpful to use a slow cooker—small or large—to keep foods warm for serving or to use as extra "oven space." We frequently use slow cookers to keep mashed potatoes warm.
2. Not all slow cookers are created equal. Slow cooker brands and models vary in heat temperature. Don't assume that a new or different slow cooker will require the same cooking time as another. It is helpful to test a new slow cooker recipe for timing before you make it for a crowd.
3. Look for a programmable slow cooker that has a manual setting for temperature and time. Some slow cookers automatically change to the warm setting after a set number of hours. This is a great feature, but as you know, you may have to adjust the cooking time and you don't want to be locked into cooking for longer than needed.
4. Use a meat thermometer. A common problem with slow cookers is dry and overcooked meat. Remember, the size of a roast or chicken makes a big difference with timing. A meat thermometer is a helpful tool to check for doneness. Aim for 160° for beef and 170° for poultry. NOTE: Try using bone-in meats in your slow cooker. We find that they turn out juicier than their boneless counterparts.
5. Use your slow cooker for many of your favorite recipes. You don't have to use a specific recipe to use your slow cooker; you can adapt many of your favorite recipes. Chili is a favorite recipe to make in a slow cooker. After the meat is browned, place it and the remaining ingredients in the slow cooker on low for 4-6 hours. Use this same technique for a variety of your favorite soup or stew recipes. NOTE: Plan ahead! It's easier to cut/trim meat, chop vegetables and measure spices the night before. Place in the refrigerator so they can be quickly put in the slow cooker in the morning.
6. Shredded pork is another easy recipe to make. Simply place a 3-4 pound pork loin roast in your slow cooker with ½ cup water, ½ cup apple cider vinegar, salt, pepper, and tabasco sauce (to taste). After cooking on low for 7-8 hours, cut meat across the grain and shred it with a fork. Serve with coleslaw or Mediterranean Potato Salad (p. 121).
7. Come home to a delicious, tender chicken. You can roast a whole chicken in the slow cooker while you are at work during the day. Simply brush the outside of the bird with butter, sprinkle with salt and pepper, and fill the cavity with pieces of onion, celery and carrot. You can add poultry seasoning or another favorite seasoning. Cook on low for about 8 hours. You will love the end product!
8. Winter squash or baked potatoes work well in the slow cooker. Simply poke a few holes in the skin and place the squash or potatoes in your slow cooker with about one-half cup of water.

Cook on low for about 4 hours—it's that easy! Add some butter and salt to the squash; put sour cream or butter on the baked potato. Yum!

9. Don't overfill your slow cooker. Most manufacturers recommend filling no more than two-thirds of the pot to ensure that the food cooks thoroughly.

Try these tips and discover how your slow cooker can be your time-saving, go-to solution for preparing meals. Not sure where to start? Try the Instant Pot Citrus Pork (p. 76), Crock Pot® Chuck Roast (p. 53), or Chili (p. 52) recipes in this book.

How to Hard Boil Eggs

1. In a saucepan, bring 6 cups of water to a boil.
2. Using a spoon, gently place eggs in the water.
3. Lower the heat to low and simmer for 9 minutes.
4. Remove from heat and rinse under cold water.
5. Peel and eat or refrigerate.

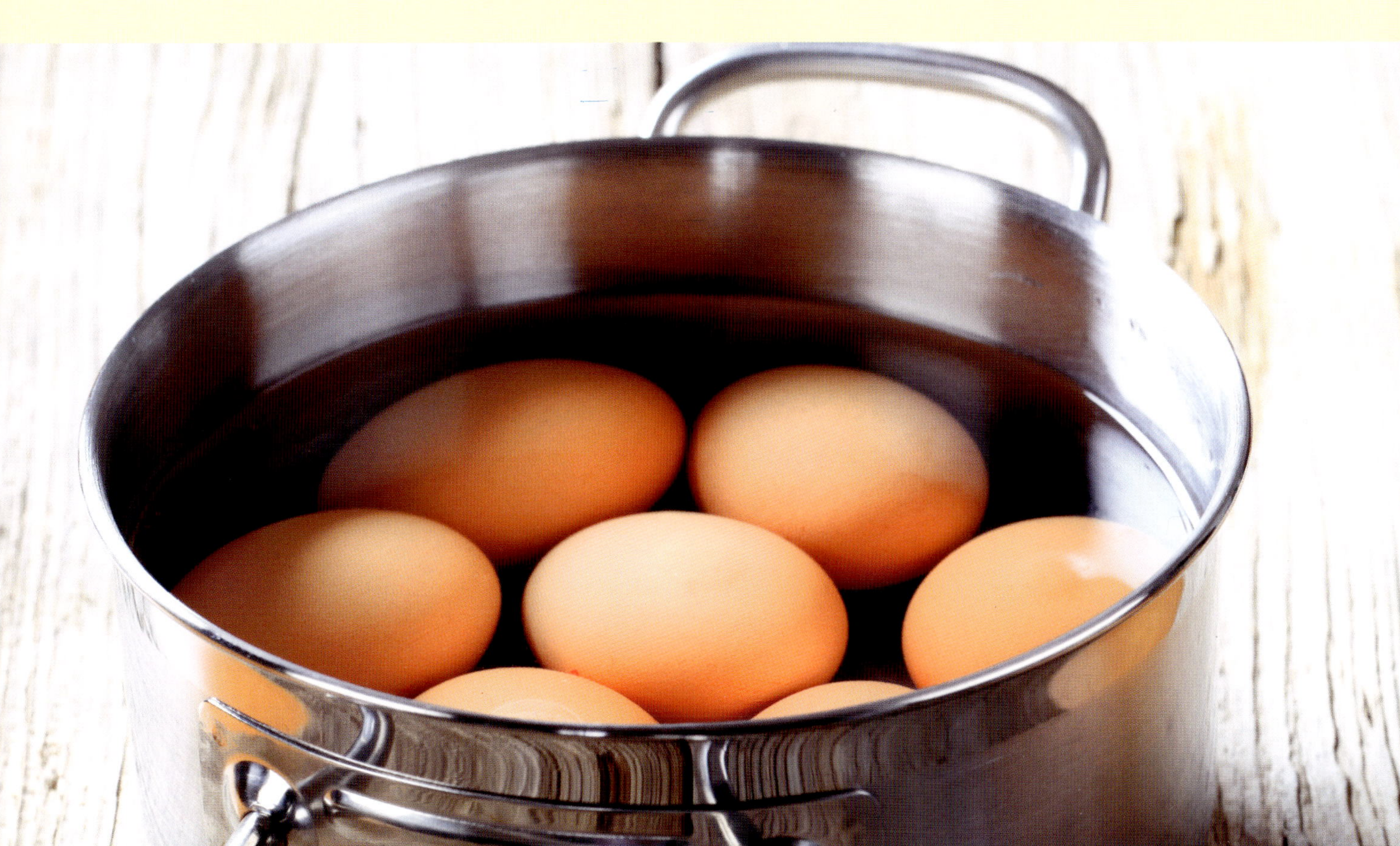

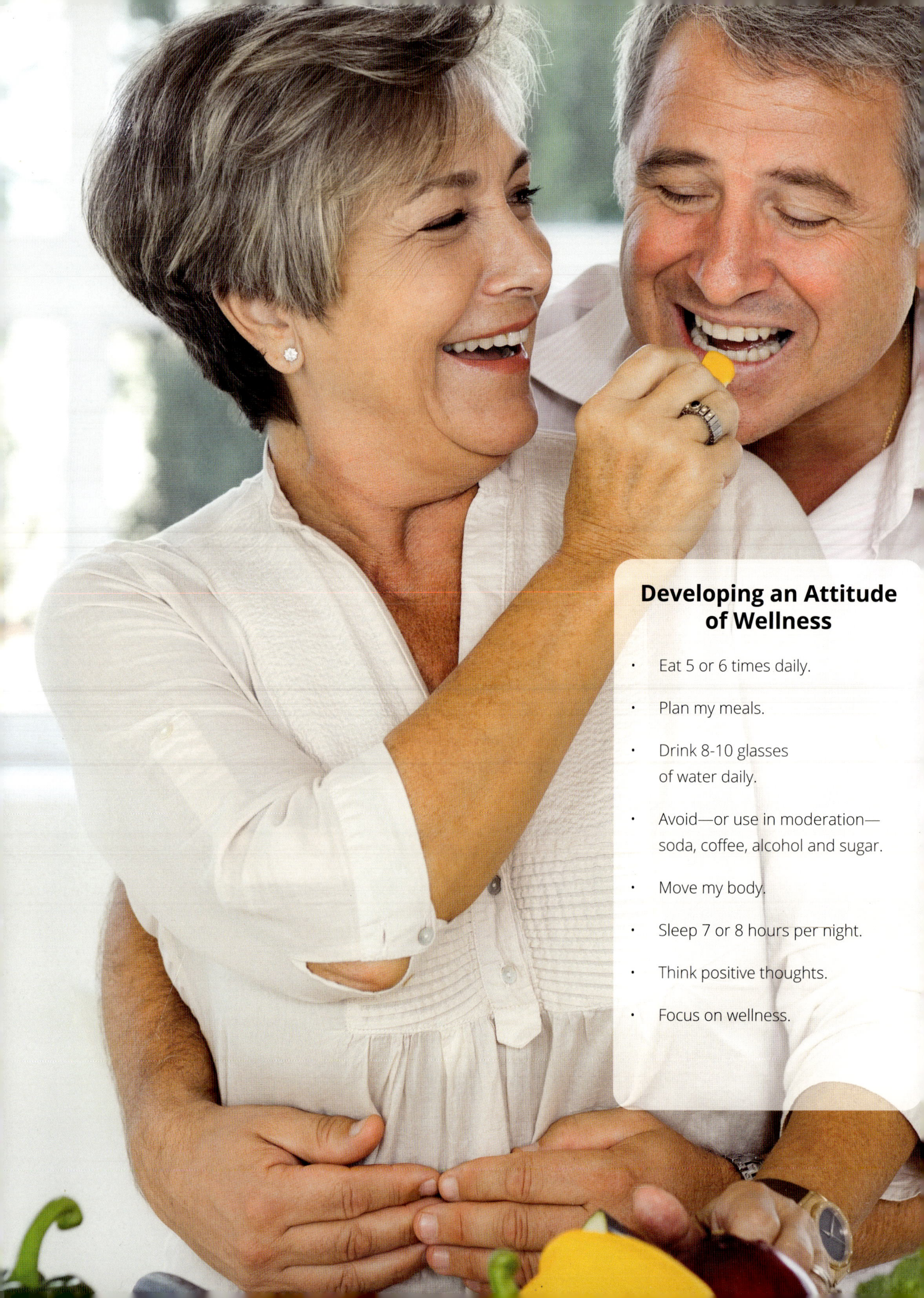

Developing an Attitude of Wellness

- Eat 5 or 6 times daily.
- Plan my meals.
- Drink 8-10 glasses of water daily.
- Avoid—or use in moderation—soda, coffee, alcohol and sugar.
- Move my body.
- Sleep 7 or 8 hours per night.
- Think positive thoughts.
- Focus on wellness.